child safety is no accident

A Parents' Handbook of Emergencies

child safety is no accident

A Parents' Handbook of Emergencies

authored by

Jay M. Arena, M.D.
Miriam Bachar, M.S.

duke university press
durham, north carolina

Second Printing, 1979
© 1978, Duke University Press
L.C.C. card number 77-80346
I.S.B.N. 0-8223-0390-6

PREFACE

Children today face risks, never experienced by previous generations, because of advancing technology which both enriches and endangers our lives.

The purpose of this book is threefold: to provide parents, teachers, and others who have responsibility for the growth and development of children with (1) guidance on how to develop a safe and satisfying family life style for children; (2) information on how to prevent accidents through sensible precautions; and (3) experience-tested, first aid techniques to use immediately when an accident or illness requiring emergency treatment occurs.

Because of increasing medical and health care demands, vital members of the health team for the care of children are parents and others who, even though they may have no professional medical training, are charged with protecting the welfare of children. A large part of health care responsibility rests on the shoulders of these people. They are first level health care evaluators who must make the decision as to whether children in their care should be given professional medical treatment. Yet, little is being done to inform parents and others about how to do this job.

Parents and other responsible adults must see themselves as captains of the child health team, using their physician as coach. They must learn to instill good safety habits in children, and to administer basic first aid care. They need to gain confidence through knowledge for handling the many child ailments and accidents that inevitably occur. Parents need to know when to call for professional medical help and how to take care of the situation until such help is reached.

Although this book can be used as a quick reference in an emergency situation, it is also designed for study. Study the table of contents; together with the comprehensive Index, it can be invaluable when you have a problem and need to use the book. Learn the basic principles and techniques in this book and you will be able to provide for the safety and well-being of children, from birth on through their early teens.

Our special thanks go to Dr. Donald A. Cornely, Chairman of the Department of Maternal and Child Health, Johns Hopkins University. Dr. Cornely read and commented on the manuscript during its preparation, offering constructive professional suggestions as well as helpful encouragement to the authors.

J.M.A.

M.B.

CONTENTS

PART FIVE Ready Reference Guide

PART ONE

Attitudes and Life Styles

INTRODUCTION

Accidents are the number one health hazard for children. More than one-third of childhood deaths between the ages of one and fourteen are caused by accidents, which kill more children than the five leading fatal diseases combined. Accidents are not only the largest single cause of death in children under fifteen years of age, but also are the leading cause of disability, permanent or temporary, in those over the age of one year.

How can we reduce the number of accidents and achieve a greater level of safety for our children?

For reasons that remain unclear, we tend to ignore or to be indifferent to many kinds of potentially dangerous circumstances. Auto accidents result in tragically large numbers of deaths and injuries each year. As a society we continue to put up with these impersonal statistics and tragic events. Gun control receives attention because of the deaths of prominent public officials; yet the deaths of more than 500 children a year as a result of gun accidents do not seem to have much impact on the public.

As parents, we give affection and protection to a child. We place an enormous value on that child's life, on the healthy and safe way in which it is lived and experienced. As individuals, we can and must take more effective action to assure the safety of our children.

Parents, teachers, day-care center workers, camp personnel and others who are responsible for children need to be aware of dangers specific to distinct stages of child growth and development. Knowing what the most likely causes of accident may be at certain ages will help all of us anticipate such situations and, forearmed with knowledge, prevent or reduce their occurrence.

Most of the things we do with our children that affect safety can be grouped under four approaches or ways of intervening:

- protection
- discipline
- regulation
- teaching

Protection means preventing the child and the potential hazard from interacting—sharp knives are out of reach; wall sockets are covered; a toddler's hand is held when crossing the street.

Discipline means firmly and justifiably expecting obedience—touching the stove is not allowed; leaving the yard is not permitted without first asking.

Regulation means guiding behavior through discipline and mutual understanding. Your child's behavior should be expected to vary with age, experience, and surroundings—leaving the yard is permitted so that a four-year-old may go to a neighbor's yard *on the same side of the street*; a nine-year-old is permitted to visit a friend who lives three blocks away *but must return home at a specific time.*

Teaching means sharing information and suggesting ways of using it—bicycle riders must follow specific rules of the road; a first-grader should know how to take care of himself going to and from school.

We can work more effectively toward avoiding accidents by associating our child's age with a particular way of intervening. It is important to be aware of how to use different kinds of intervention so that you can develop the capability to use them in the proper relationship to your child's stage of growth and development.

For the infant, *absolute protection is essential*. Gradually this must be reduced and replaced by increasing amounts of teaching, discipline, and regulation. Most often, as your children grow, you will be using not one type of intervention but two or more in proper combination or sequence.

Thus, we may describe our goal as an attempt to consider and deal with accident prevention for children through a coordinated approach which takes into consideration:

- the age of our child
- the hazards that our child is most likely to encounter
- the type of intervention we need to employ which is most effective

To achieve this coordinated approach will require some planning with serious thinking, experimenting, learning, and teaching on your part; but just as other things that you do with and for your children are learned and become automatic and spontaneous, so also will you need to incorporate safe habits into the family's natural life styles. You must make safe behavior patterns part of your children's lives. The result should be a way of life which quite easily and routinely enhances your children's safety.

We do not imply that all accidents can be eliminated. Each of us must accept the human fate of surviving in a dangerous world and realize that accidents—often tragic ones—can happen because of circumstances beyond our control. But focusing attention on achieving safety for your children can help prevent accidents. Be forewarned and forearmed with the proper information.

The information contained in this book is offered as self-education as well as a reference for the examination of your own everyday activities as well as those of your child. Safety for your child can be accomplished only within the context of the times in which we live. Today's hazards are more complex than ever before—and yet we cannot withdraw from them. We can cope effectively with them if we learn and use the essential elements of safety.

SAFETY HABITS AND ACCIDENT PREVENTION   1

Safety in Today's World

If our lives never changed, we could try perhaps to make a list of "dangerous situations and dangerous objects." Then we might try to provide a prescription on how to anticipate a particular danger under a specific set of circumstances; and how to intervene at the propitious moment and avoid the hazard. However, life is ever-changing, and the times in which we live are fast-paced, with technology improving our lives, but also often threatening our very existence. Daily, our children are confronted with challenges which we as children never experienced. Admonitions of "do this" or "don't do that," can be outdated quickly. In this book, you will find many "do's" and "don'ts." But there is no substitute for intelligent action based on understanding of the emergency that confronts you.

Most of us do the best we can for our children out of natural love and concern. The complexity of life today, however, is such that we need to be informed about its danger to life and limb. "Professionals" are giving us more and more information about specific products—car seats which we should buy to protect our child, toys which are safe to play with, locking devices which we can utilize to keep harmful substances out of reach of our children. Through TV and radio, newspapers, magazines, and books, we are exposed to safety advice each day. Hundreds of items of published information about fire hazards, water safety, pedestrian accidents, and a host of other specific accidents are available from a variety of sources. But basically we need to develop an understanding of the predictable patterns and events which regularly occur in all our children's lives.

We can identify characteristics of our family life style or pattern of living. We also can recognize our child's pattern of growth and development. Even though we may know these things only in a general way, we can take advantage of their predictability and introduce more effective safety models.

In considering how to improve safety for our children, we must think about three factors which often lead to an accident:

1. The child as we identify him in terms of his age or stage of growth and development.
2. The physical and social situation in which the child is at the given time of the potential or actual accident.
3. The event that is emerging, or about to occur.

For example, we have a two-year-old, just placed in a bathtub by his mother, when the telephone rings. Should she leave a child of this age alone in the bathtub while she answers the phone? How different for a six-month-old? . . . a four-year-old?

For each age group there are identifiable circumstances and responses which are often associated with children's accidents. These include:

- Hunger or fatigue (particularly during the hour before a scheduled meal, during late afternoon, or before bedtime)
- Hyperactivity
- Illness, pregnancy, or menstruation of the mother

Safety Habits and Accident Prevention   7

- Recent substitution of a person caring for a child (as from mother to sister)
- Continually tense relationships between parents
- Illness or death of other family members, taking most of the mother's attention
- Sudden change of a child's environment (moving from one residence to another or at vacation time)
- Mother rushed or too busy (Saturday is the worst accident day, particularly between 3:00 and 6:00 p.m.)
- Parental lack of understanding of what to expect at various stages in childhood development

Most of the things you do result in events which have either little or no accident potential; but some can lead to events with high accident potential. Tipping the balance in favor of occasions with little or no accident potential is the goal you should strive for.

Planning a Safe Living Pattern

Before you can begin to do something in a different way, you must take a few minutes to think about how you and your children do things now. Some people are quick and eager to try anything. Others are more deliberate and consider the consequences before acting. Others are unsure and reluctant to consider new things. Life would not be possible if all potentially dangerous events were to disappear. However, some family life styles overprotect children; others unnecessarily expose them to danger.

A safe life style does not mean a total absence of hazards, nor does it mean constant restrictions, limitations, or nagging cautions. A safe life style exists when you are aware of the inevitable hazards in life and, through knowledge and good safety habits, feel that you can cope with them under extraordinary situations.

Appropriate attention to safety by you and your child will strengthen your child's courage and his ability to take risks and enjoy adventures. He will learn to anticipate hazards and to remain in control of his reactions to them. His safety will not be dependent upon external controls but will become a part of his developing life style.

Attitudes About Accident Prevention

An accident can be a sudden, unexpected event which may result in injury or death. It is important, however, to be aware of the fact that accidents are not always due to chance or to events beyond our control. Accidents are complex, often the result of a complicated interrelation-ship of factors, of which human performance is only one. Within the context of daily living it is possible for you to look at some of the factors which lead to accidents. You can make practical changes in your life style which can result in fewer accidents.

Start with an appreciation of safety which can become a part of your way of life. Regard for safety grows out of deep-seated values and concerns. An infant continually experiences your complete caring for him. From this care, the child learns gradually to care for himself and for others, and begins to feel that he is worth taking care of. He learns to behave responsibly and safely because he values himself as well as others. To be loved is to be cared about and cared for, to be protected and kept safe. As your child grows in responsibility, he learns that to love or have a friend is also to respect and care about that person's well-being. A commitment to helping your child grow with good safety habits is to instill in him values that encourage independent action—and yet with full respect for the safety of others.

While your child is learning about love and respect, he is growing in many other ways. He is becoming aware of the words you use. He begins to listen and repeat what you say. All children learn to speak the language they hear, whether it is English or Chinese or French. They learn to speak the language of the adults around them. Just as children learn to speak the complex languages of their cultures, so too can they learn to behave safely if the adults around them make safety information available and, more importantly, set the example. This information should be offered in many forms. It will be offered through the expectations you have about how you want your children to dress, eat, play, obey. It will be offered when your child watches you drive, play, swim, walk. He will soon compare what you say with what you do.

Children must be allowed to explore and learn. Rather than trying to discourage these natural desires and needs, you should help your children develop the ability to cope with new, sometimes hazardous, situations. If you adopt this attitude, your innate common sense plus your special awareness of your child can be brought together for safer living.

Habits of Accident Prevention

Our lives are filled with innumerable efforts to deal with unglamorous events that may be dull and repetitious. We understand and accept the responsibility for the routines needed to avoid and prevent undesirable events: every day we dress to avoid discomfort; eat to avoid hunger; rest to avoid fatigue; build friendships to avoid loneliness. We know that the rewards of such daily repetitive actions are difficult to identify each time. But we do recognize a sense of comfort and well-being which is our motivation for continuing to repeat these actions.

Safety must be understood to require that same motivation. Safety actions must become just as important as those many other routine chores we have learned to accept as contributing to our pleasure and comfort.

You are doing many repetitive things now which prevent injury to the infant you cradle in your arms, supporting his head until his muscles become stronger; the toddler whose hand you hold when crossing the street; the school child you remind to obey his teacher.

Habits of accident prevention should be thought of as normal daily living practices. Until these practices become automatic, a specific review of how you try to avoid accidents and what your child does is needed. In order to change and improve behavior, think about what you are doing now. Habits generally fall into three categories:

1. Your behavior habits which children observe and absorb, with very little, if any, awareness on your part.
2. The pattern of ways in which you respond to your children when they actively seek some interchange with you.
3. The manner in which you direct and teach your children.

LEARNING ABOUT SAFETY

2

Learning Through Casual Observation

What you do demonstrates safe or unsafe methods to your child. An enormous amount of safety education occurs indirectly. Become more conscious of this and try to modify some of the things you do. At the same time, remain confident and relaxed about assessing your own habits. Your family pattern is made up of a variety of practical arrangements, both physical and emotional, with which you are psychologically comfortable. These arrangements are also the setting in which the greatest efforts toward accident prevention have to take place.

You arrange your kitchen or work area for your convenience in doing the job. It detracts little, if at all, by incorporating safety ideas. Consider how the items you arrange make it easier to deal with a potentially dangerous situation. Most important, consider how the safety ideas you put to use make you feel comfortable and allow you to deal with your child in a relaxed manner, a convenient, comfortable manner which capitalizes on your intuition and enables you to put to use valuable facts.

Learning Through Casual Interchange

How you respond to your child must grow out of an awareness of what response is appropriate for his age, his physical and emotional needs, as well as your expectations about him. Your responses can follow a pattern with which you are comfortable, but you must be flexible. You must remember that a child is subject to stresses, opportunity or lack of it, and rewards or lack of them. The nature of the learning machinery varies from child to child.

We frequently make one of two mistakes in teaching our children. We either credit a child with more mental capability than he possesses or we assume he is unable to think for himself. In both situations we fail to appreciate that we are dealing with a mind and body in constant development and change. Parents and adults who work with children must anticipate the continuing changes, the various stages of growth and development.

The physical care and love you give your child establishes the basic communication. When the toddler brings a flower or the older child asks a question, you have the opportunity to continue a pattern of communication between you and your children. This continuing communication throughout the child's life, as expressed through your attention and affection, is one of the most important tools you have to enhance safety.

Chances of getting hurt grow as the child grows, although the circumstances may differ. Hazards multiply as the baby learns to creep, walk, climb, and explore. Often accidents occur when you are not aware of your child's physical and mental capabilities at a specific stage of development. You are out of tune with your child's needs and growth.

Many parents believe that a warning or punishment is sufficient to stop a pre-school child from getting into trouble; but most pre-school children don't remember explanations, may not remember warnings, and often don't connect disciplinary action with the behavior that prompts it. For example, a four-year-old, named Mary, was told by her mother that if she went into the street she would be spanked. Instead of looking for the real danger, Mary walked into the street looking back over her shoulder to see if her mother was watching. That was the reason she didn't see the car that struck her. Mary had never been warned, "If you go into the street, you may be hit by a car." Mary had never been taught that cars are a hazard; all she had ever worried about was a spanking.

After an accident, parents frequently make remarks like, "I never realized Lynn could reach the top of the stove," or "I had no idea Mike could crawl up all the stairs." As hard as it is to anticipate and keep up with a child's rapid physical and mental growth, you must do just that in order to protect your child from accidents, and provide development of good health habits.

Learning Through Specific Teaching

Let us consider some general principles about how you can go about sharing your safety knowledge with your children. First, you need to spend some time considering your child's needs in relationship to his particular stage of growth and development. Every once in a while parents have to take stock, for example, of the child's need for new clothing: What no longer fits; are those that do fit appropriate for the weather expected in the next few months; how much can you afford to spend on new clothes? Now include safety behavior in your thinking.

What you want him to understand about safety and how you expect him to behave in a safe way must be relevant to his world. As your child grows from the infant who spends a great deal of time sleeping and eating to a person who can ride a bike to school, your safety activities and expectations must change with his development.

Your child is constantly and rapidly outgrowing the environment in which you have his safety very easily under your direct control, captive in his crib or playpen or house or yard. Gradually he moves into situations where you will have less direct control, and you must begin to trust his capacity to take care of himself some of the time. Eventually you become aware that he is not captive at all: your control over what happens to him diminishes rapidly. For a time and under circumstances appropriate to his age, you offer indirect control through restrictions:

"You may play outside in front of the house or at Billy's house, but you may not cross the street."

Later on, the restriction/control arrangements may be changed:

"You may ride your bike after school but you must be home by 4:30."

For older children, the restriction/control arrangements may or may not be discussed, and are often indirect and implied:

"What time will you be home from the basketball game?"

Left to the older child's discretion are matters of transportation to and from the game, who else may be going that you know, and other information both parent and child have incorporated into their behavior and family pattern.

What is taking place over the time span from captive infant to responsible adolescent? The child begins very early to learn that he is gradually assuming control over more of his own behavior in increasingly complex situations. He begins to understand that he has responsibility for what happens to himself beginning with just a few minutes hence and building to an awareness of a more distant time. For example, you may tell your five-year-old:

"I am going next door to borrow some sugar. Stay out

of the kitchen or you may burn yourself on the hot oven."

He begins to consider the consequences of his actions and learns to act accordingly. These heartening achievements and conditioning are the rewards, for the child and his family, of your repeated efforts to guide, encourage and teach him.

Relating Safety Habits to Reality

Activities which are geared to the development of safe behavior must fall within the framework of the child's as well as the adult's experience—family, neighborhood, and school. You should make sure that your perception of your child's environment is not too different from that of his own. For example, do you know enough about the sitters you leave him with? As the child grows, are you sufficiently aware of the school environment so that you can offer guidance to your child about his safety there? What are the attitudes and customs of the neighborhood in which he plays? Do you know which families leave guns around the house? How about the person with whom you share a car pool? Is your child safe with that driver?

Do not overlook the need to consider your child's own view of himself as a person. Just as he grows and changes physically, his thoughts about himself change. Safe behavior can best be accomplished as part of a sense of self-worth and a desire to take care of oneself. You must understand the child's strengths and weaknesses, help him overcome his self-doubts, share in his accomplishments. Be sensitive to his awareness of himself, how he believes he fits into the times in which he lives, and what he understands the family and society expects of him.

Your child should be learning to relate the safe behavior used in your presence to other and stranger environments. Toddlers are notorious for getting into cabinets, medicine chests, dressers. Serious and fatal poisonings are most frequent between one and three years of age. Many parents take extra care to keep poisonous substances out of reach, *but forget to consider what their child may do when he is in some other home where such substances are accessible.*

Research studies have shown that locking away poisonous substances has not entirely eliminated the problem. Does grandma lock everything up? How about a playmate's mother? In addition to keeping dangerous things out of reach, you must help your children learn better self-control.

There is no reason small children should be allowed access to all closets, drawers, cabinets. Some should be off limits even though dangerous items are not kept there. You should allow the child freedom to explore, but not freedom to abuse your own needs for order and privacy. If it is acceptable to you, let the toddler play on the floor with your pots. If it is not acceptable, provide firm, consistent restriction. Along with, "No, you may not," and when physically removing a young child, you should include information about why the restriction is necessary. "You may not take anything out of the kitchen cabinets, but you may ask me for something you might like to use," is an appropriate restriction for a three-year-old. "You may use only unbreakable cups when you get yourself some milk," is a fair restriction for a five-year-old.

A child must be taught to begin to make judgments appropriate to his age. He must learn to reason rather than simply react emotionally. A child who can resist playmates whose suggestions for play activities are dangerous will be learning early an attitude important for the rest of his life.

You help your child make appropriate judgments by

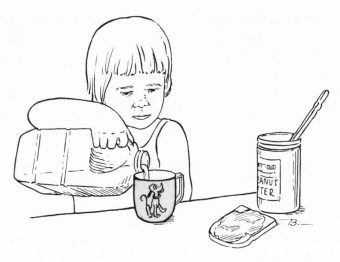

"You may use only unbreakable cups when you get yourself some milk," is a fair restriction for a five-year-old.

the way in which you deal with one specific situation about safe behavior, but can also extend the specific correction to include a general discussion of safety principles. When a neighbor calls to complain that your eight-year-old has climbed her fence and trampled some favorite roses, your reprimand to the child may be limited to a discussion of the specific wrongdoing. Or, beyond that, what do fences mean? Sometimes they are used to protect something of particular personal value. Othertimes, fences are used to restrict people from severe danger: an electrical power station, railroad tracks, a swimming pool, an abandoned quarry. While being asked to be more considerate of what is important to your neighbor, the child can be reminded to think about the self-discipline required to respect all fences, whatever their purpose.

In sum:

1. Teach the child to distinguish between the risks he may take and those he should avoid.

2. Teach him the best way of dealing with those dangers that cannot be avoided.
3. Teach him discipline and obedience. Discipline is setting limits through education, parental example, encouragement, cooperation, insistence, temporary isolation if necessary, and sometimes punishment.

Hazard Clusters

Part of the reason accidents continue to cause large numbers of deaths and injuries in spite of intense and varied safety campaigns is that people find it very difficult to absorb safety information and put it to practical use. The information remains isolated from family life and is soon forgotten.

We suggest you begin to think about possible hazards in two broad categories or clusters:

1. Product-directed circumstances where the *proper use of something* is the key to whether the situation will be safe or unsafe. For example, electrical appliances, firearms, laundry bleach, matches, all can be considered safe when properly used but hazardous and sometimes fatal when used improperly. All products have characteristics intrinsic to their function which can be dangerous. You should know what these dangers are and then apply that knowledge to maintain safety during the product's use. An electric saw, an ax, a carving knife, all are designed to cut. Only children whose physical ability and intelligence are developed enough to recognize these dangers and avoid them should be taught how to use these tools.

2. People-directed circumstances where *behavior* is the key to whether the situation will be safe or unsafe. For example, proper behavior contributes to safety with animals, at school, as a pedestrian; and improper behavior

does not. Self-discipline, courtesy, and obedience to certain rules, laws, or customs serve to maintain the balance for safety. Feeding wild or stray animals, running at school, darting between parked cars upsets the balance and increases hazard potential. The safety of a two-year-old in the bathtub is dependent on the behavior of the mother.

Thus, we can try to consider groups of hazards whose similarities suggest that a primary focus must be on *use* or on *behavior*. Consider again what has been said earlier about the child's age—the need to understand the particular hazards specific to distinct stages of growth and development. Also, we have discussed ways in which we are likely to intervene as we try to anticipate and reduce the occurrence of accidents: we have suggested that most of the things can be grouped under four approaches—protection; discipline; regulation; and teaching.

A Safety Concept

We now can bring together our understanding of the child's age, the appropriate intervention process, and an identification of whether the hazard focus is primarily on use or behavior.

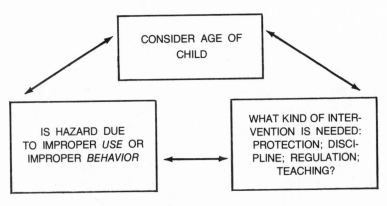

We have available, then, a triangular concept about safety which may enable us to make effective use of information now and in the future. As new products come on the market and as new situations are encountered by the child, we can consider where they will fit into our particular program of child safety.

In the following material about specific ages and hazards we will include suggestions about which focus—**use** or **behavior**—seems most likely to lead to a prevention program that will be basic and effective.

PART TWO

**Stages of Growth and Development:
Hazards and Avoidance**

INTRODUCTION

Safety habits must begin as early in the child's life as possible. Start now with your newborn; but even with older children it is never too late. "Average developmental stages" are discussed throughout this book. Remember that a child is not necessarily slow or abnormal if he cannot perform all the activities mentioned for his age group. If you have questions or concerns, you should consult your physician.

For each age group, we will discuss some of the more common hazards as well as those which cause the greatest number of deaths and permanent injury. Consider that one cannot list or discuss beforehand every possible event which may pose a threat to your child. The basic ideas you should keep in mind to help you handle unforeseen situations include:

1. The age of the child and his relative ability to function on his own.
2. Your family's life style, or pattern of living.
3. The nature of the potential hazard.
4. Your way of helping your child deal with the hazard threat.

FROM BIRTH TO TWELVE MONTHS

3

Suffocation, falls, poisonings, drownings, and burns cause more deaths to infants from birth to twelve months than all diseases combined.

Birth to Four Months

Newborn babies are completely helpless and require complete and constant protection. For a month or so after birth, the baby's head will flip forward or flop backward if not supported. By the end of the first month the normal infant shows selective regard for his mother's face. At the age of two months, he follows her moving fingers with his eyes. At the third month, he can crudely manipulate a rattle.

The basic activities of the infant are eating, being changed of soiled diapers, being bathed, and sleeping. What could be safer! But, unfortunately, there are many dangers, even in the apparent safety of your home.

To safeguard an infant from accidents, it is vital to observe rigorously three basic rules:

1. Never underestimate the rapid rate of baby's physical and mental development. It increases, literally, while your back is turned.
2. Always be alert for the unexpected.
3. Never leave a baby alone outside the confined areas of a crib or playpen when he is awake.

Feeding

Since infants derive great pleasure from feeding, they put everything into their mouths as soon as they can pick up objects. Mothers constantly must be on the alert to *keep out of the baby's reach small objects* such as pins, buttons, nuts, and hard candy that can cause death by choking if they are swallowed.

During feeding, hold the baby in your arms instead of propping the bottle. Some infants spit up and then inhale milk or other liquids. Make sure that the nipple opening of the bottle is not too large. If the baby does start to gag, remove the bottle and, after he has fully regained his breath, begin again. Never feed your baby while you are lying in bed (some mothers do this when breastfeeding at night); you might doze off and roll over on the baby.

The first cardinal rule—*never underestimate the rapid rate of a baby's physical development*—is particularly important at about three months. A mother who never has seen her baby turn over may think it is safe to leave the child for a moment on a table or a bassinet while she reaches for a diaper or a can of talcum powder. At that precise moment the baby may turn over for the first time and roll off the table, an accident that kills scores of infants every year and leaves many more with permanent disabling injuries.

Since infants differ in temperament and activity (some are constantly wiggling!), it is wise to form the habit of *never leaving your baby unguarded on anything from which he might fall*. Make it a habit to take your baby with you if you must reach for anything which prevents you from keeping at least one protective hand on him.

If you have to answer the door or the telephone while you are in the middle of a diaper change or a bath, wrap your baby up and take him with you or put him back in the crib with the sides up. (Of course, you can ignore that

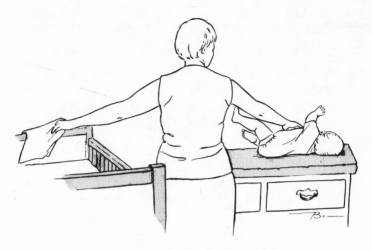

Keep a protective hand on your child.

telephone call! If it's important, the caller will try again.) An unexpected visitor or phone call often turns out to last much longer than intended.

Changing Diapers

Falls to the floor by infants from tables, couches, or beds used for changing diapers happen too frequently. No matter what area or equipment you use for changing diapers, you should construct some kind of barrier to prevent your baby from falling. For example, some diaper changing tables have a safety strap which fastens across the child's chest or stomach. The strap should be checked to see that it will not slip or break. If your baby is being changed on a couch or an adult bed, a barrier can be created by folding blankets or large towels and placing one on either side of the infant. Or you can construct your own strap arrangement by folding a length of any sturdy material which is not harsh on the baby's body to a width of approximately three inches. For use on a bed, make the material long enough so that the "strap" will go under as well as over the mattress and can be tied across the baby's chest or stomach. When not using the bed for changing diapers, simply tuck the "strap" under the edges of the mattress for use the next time. The same kind of "strap" can be made for use on a couch with cushions, going under and over the cushion, tying across the infant, and storing under the cushion after use.

Bathing

Check the temperature of the bath water with your elbow to determine proper temperature. The water should feel comfortably warm—not hot or cold. *Don't leave the baby alone in the bath for any reason*, since it takes

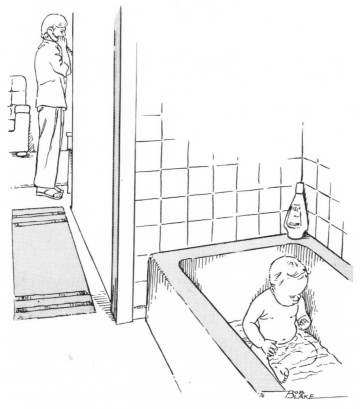

Don't ever leave the baby alone during his bath for any reason.

only seconds to drown. Always keep one hand on the baby during the bath, and wrap him up and take him with you if you must answer the phone or doorbell.

Your baby is more safely bathed in something smaller than the bathtub—the washbasin, kitchen sink, bathinette, or small plastic tub. Use only a small amount of water at first until you get the knack of holding the baby securely. A basin or tub is less slippery if you line the bottom with a diaper or bath towel. Hold the baby firmly so that his head is supported on your wrist, and with the fingers of that hand hold him securely in his armpit.

Do you smoke? Never do so while carrying the baby. The infant may grab for the lighted end. Hot ashes can cause skin and eye burns.

High Chairs and Seats

Seats for babies should never be placed on table tops or other high surfaces. Be imaginative in protecting your child. Use dog leash hooks to fasten gates and even harnesses that restrain a child in a high chair. Small fingers and inexperience will soon give up attempting to deal with that mystery. Remember: either hold your baby or confine him when you must do an "out of sight" chore.

Toys

Toys should be too large to swallow, too tough to break, and without sharp or hard edges. At this early stage in the infant's development, your baby will enjoy toys to look at and listen to, such as a mobile firmly fastened above the crib or carriage out of his reach; sturdy, nonflammable rattles, bells, music boxes, and brightly colored hanging toys. But be sure that the infant cannot strangle himself on the strings from which toys are suspended.

Be sure that older brothers and sisters understand

what they can safely share with the baby. Your ten-year-old must learn that his favorite marbles are not appropriate for the infant. A toddler must learn that the baby is not a plaything but a fragile person like himself who needs care and protection.

Four to Seven Months

A particularly dangerous period in the infant's development begins about four months after birth.

Babies begin to turn over by themselves, usually from the stomach to the back, and expose themselves to a common cause of fatality in their first year—*mechanical suffocation*. Covers, pillows, and articles of clothing left in the crib or playpen may accidentally fall on your baby's face. At this stage, the infant's movements are too feeble and uncoordinated to throw off the obstruction to his breathing. Death can result in a few terrifying moments.

To avert such accidents, all objects that can be dislodged by a baby's movements should be kept out of the sleeping area. *A firm mattress* also should be used to make sure your baby's face does not burrow into it too deply.

At four months, the average infant prefers to lie on his back, lifts his head and shoulders, and can roll from side to back or back to side. He holds his head erect when carried, pushes his feet against the floor and reaches for objects.

At five months, he can pick up a toy on manual contact and can roll over, almost always at first from stomach to back.

At six months, the infant prefers to sit up with support, can roll from back to stomach and vice versa, uses his hands to reach, grasp, crumble and bang objects, and uses his thumb in grasping a cup.

At seven months, he can sit alone, grab things, and is able to push up to hand-knee creeping posture.

The infant of 4-7 months still needs full-time protection. Accidents are more frequent than in the first three months because the child grasps now and moves more. Since your baby can now turn over by himself, he should not be left alone on a bed, couch, or table, even for a second. The combination of learning to grasp things and putting everything in his mouth can be deadly.

As soon as he can sit up, your baby will be safer in his highchair, carriage, stroller, and infant seat *when he is wearing a harness.* A playpen can be a safe place for you to put the baby when you are busy. It also offers the infant an opportunity for movement and play.

In choosing a playpen, keep in mind how much space your child will need, where the playpen will be placed, how easily it can be moved and, above all, how sturdily it is constructed. If you choose a wooden playpen, make sure the side slats are set close enough together so that your baby can't get his head caught between them. Be certain that the paint finish is lead-free and smooth enough so that the child won't get splinters or scratch himself. If you buy a mesh playpen, check the openings in the netting to see that they aren't so wide that arms or legs can be poked through and get caught: be sure that any metal catches on the pen are outside the railing. *Never tie toys to a playpen railing:* a child could strangle himself on the string.

Keep playpens in areas that can be readily observed and away from potentially dangerous objects such as lamps, cords, glass, venetian blinds, fireplace tools, and the stove. Make sure there are no electrical outlets within reach.

When your baby learns to crawl and creep, you should barricade the tops and bottoms of your staircases. One of the most frequent accidents to babies at the crawling stage is

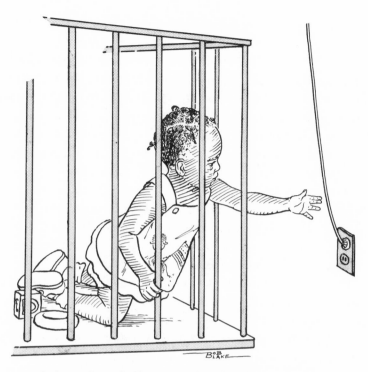

A playpen is a safe place to put the baby when you are busy.
Make sure there are no electrical outlets within reach.

falling down stairs. Babies learn to go up the stairs before they learn to go down safely. Inexpensive safety gates are available in many stores, or you may be able to construct a barrier yourself that cannot be moved easily by your child.

Keep buttons, beads, sharp objects, pins, tacks, razor blades, knives, scissors, sewing kits, hairpins, and the like safely out of a child's reach. Remember that your baby can find the smallest pin on the cleanest floor: *and he'll put it in his mouth!*

Stay in tune with your baby's world: get down on your hands and knees and crawl where he does. You may be amazed at the "deadly treasures" you can find. What has rolled under the dresser? Have you looked under your couch lately? You may discover nails or exposed springs that are in just the right location to poke into your crawler's eye.

Keep highchairs and playpens away from the stove and work counters. Keep hot liquids, hot foods, and electric cords of irons, toasters, and coffee pots out of your baby's reach. *Don't let your baby crawl around in the kitchen area during times of cooking or serving meals.* If you have space, bring the playpen into the kitchen. Some families use a low barricade at the kitchen doorway to exclude the child from the kitchen while at the same time allowing the child and mother to see and hear each other.

Place guards around heat registers in the walls or floors, and in front of fireplaces and open heaters. Be sure these guards are fastened in place so they will not fall on your child. Block off radiators and pipes with furniture wherever possible. Attractive guards can be built over radiators, but again if they have slats, be sure the slats are close enough to prevent your baby from catching his head in them. See to it that unused electric outlets are plugged or capped.

The same precautions in toys for infants (see pp. 30-31) apply for babies ages four to seven months. However, in this age group your baby will enjoy toys that he can touch, grab, squeeze, or chew on. Washable stuffed dolls or animals *without glass or button eyes* (they are cute, but dangerous); nonbreakable cups or other smooth objects to chew on; rubber or washable squeak toys; large non-breakable beads on a *strong* cord; clothespins, measuring spoons and *large* empty spools—all these fascinate a child at this age. A baby who is beginning to crawl will be intrigued by motion toys—things that roll, such as toys on wheels and large, bright balls.

But it is worth repeating—toys should be too large to swallow, too tough to break or crack, and should have no sharp edges.

Poisoning from numerous and subtle sources is a serious problem during this age. Because it will continue to be a prime cause of death and injury for the next several years of a child's life, a separate section is devoted to this topic in all its aspects: food, chemicals, and plants (see Chapter 6). Here we will simply state the basic hazards and preventive approaches.

Small children often explore by sampling things and will eat and drink anything they find, *no matter how bad it may taste*. They have little taste discrimination (children are known to eat their own feces or dog droppings).

1. Do not underestimate a child's mobility in getting to poisons.

2. Never keep household cleaners and chemicals under the sink or on low-lying shelves where your crawl-

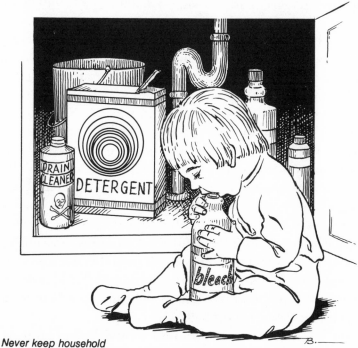

Never keep household cleaners and chemicals under the sink or on low-lying shelves where your crawling or toddling child can easily find them.

ing or toddling child can easily find them and be tempted to sample their contents. Store these items in a high cabinet (not one over a stove!) and preferably one that can be locked.

3. Dispose of empty poison containers in a safe receptacle *outside* the house where a child can't fish them out and play with them.

4. When you use medicine and household cleaners that have potentially poisonous chemicals in them, always remember to put them out of a child's reach *immediately* after using them. If the phone rings or you have to answer the door while using medicines or any household cleaners, take the bottle or container with you. Don't turn your back on a child while a poisonous substance is within his reach.

5. Don't transfer potential poisons into food containers such as bowls, jars, soft drink, or milk bottles. Many people do this unthinkingly, especially when using kerosene, turpentine, spot remover, or bleach. Youngsters innocently identify the container with a familiar drink and sometimes swallow its contents before parents can stop them.

6. Poisonous substances should *never* be stored around food. Even *you* may mistake poisons like roach powder and boric acid solution for food staples and suffer serious and fatal poisoning.

7. Be aware of *food poisoning*. Proper sterilization of a baby's formula and prompt refrigeration of milk and opened jars of baby food are extremely important habits to develop, to prevent the growth of harmful bacteria that can cause food poisoning.

Some non-poisonous food substances can be just as dangerous as poisonous ones when given to an infant by mistake: for example, putting salt instead of sugar into a baby's formula. If you transfer items such as sugar and salt to another container, be sure you **label** the new container and **read** the label before using its contents.

8. *Some plants are poisonous.* Teach your child to leave plants alone, both inside and outside the house. Many well-known decorative plants and large numbers of wild plants are poisonous. Any part of the poisonous plant —root, leaves, flowers, seeds, fruits—if swallowed may poison a child. Even nibbling on leaves, sucking on plant stalks, and drinking water in which plants have been soaking may cause poisoning.

9. *Too much medicine can be dangerous.* When giving any medication, always follow the directions on the label or, in the case of prescription drugs, the doctor's instructions. Don't make the mistake of thinking if "a little medicine is good, a lot is better." This is especially true of vitamins. One each day means just that, and not two or three. Excess vitamins can be dangerous for children and adults alike.

A Special Warning About Candy-Flavored Aspirin and Vitamins. An overdose of good-tasting medicine such as candy-flavored baby aspirin and vitamins is one of the leading causes of poisoning in young children. Children love the taste of these compounds and will climb to great heights in search of them—especially when they are hungry. Your foremost poison control policy must be: keep the aspirin and vitamins where your child cannot see and reach for them; better yet, lock them up. Do not believe that aspirin substitutes (acetaminophen) are innocuous drugs and an entirely safe substitute for aspirin. In large doses they can produce serious liver damage.

Never encourage your child to take medicine by telling him it is "candy." It is psychologically wrong, as it conditions him to think of these flavored drugs as "treats." Such misinformation has often encouraged children to search for these medicines and swallow huge and dangerous quantities of them, causing tragic poisoning.

Seven to Twelve Months

The physical changes in a child between seven and twelve months are dramatic. Your growing baby demonstrates his new capacities in many ways.

At nine months, he probably can pull up, first to his knees and then, with a hand-hold, can stand erect fairly steadily.

At ten months, most babies can stand well with almost no support at all, and can "walk" albeit unsteadily with single or double hand-hold.

At eleven months, your child may stand alone, but not for long. When he sinks to a sitting position, he can regain an erect position without assistance.

At this creeper stage, your baby's curiosity is really developing. He continues to put almost everything into his mouth, and while he has learned to pull himself up, he has also learned to pull everything else down.

Fence the staircase at the top and the bottom. Keep all matches, lighters, papers, coins, nuts, bolts, all tools and

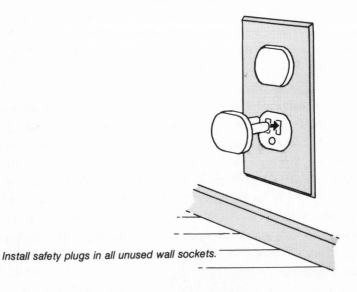

Install safety plugs in all unused wall sockets.

the like out of baby's reach. Install safety plugs in all unused wall sockets. Remove where possible easily overturned lamps; fasten electric cords securely against the wall, so that your crawler cannot yank them loose and start chewing on them. Foods on which he might choke, such as nuts of all kinds and popcorn, should be kept out of your baby's reach. Keep pails, pans, or tubs of water off the floor so baby won't fall into them—or keep your baby in his playpen or crib when you are using them. If you use baby foods that are contained in small glass jars, be extremely careful in prying off the lid so that tiny bits of glass do not chip off and fall into the jar.

Keep containers of hot food and liquids in the center of the table out of your child's reach, and keep pot handles from jutting out of the front of the stove. Hanging tablecloths can be especially dangerous, easily pulled by the child, causing everything on the table to end up on the floor and the child. Electric fans, heaters, and vaporizers should *not* be placed on the floor where your baby can get to them.

Precautions against poisoning must continue as outlined earlier (in the section about 4-7 months old) and as discussed in detail in Chapter 6. Remember: what is useful for you can be dangerous for your child. Aspirin for a headache, polish for cleaning furniture, bug spray, and laundry detergent can be child-killers.

At this stage of development, your child will love toys that he can stack and put one inside the other such as nests of blocks, boxes of different sizes and shapes, measuring spoons and cups, and colored cones. Soft, washable stuffed animals (*without button or glass eyes!*) are also fun. Stitch on facial features, if you like, before giving the toy to your child. *Caution*: Some children may be allergic to a particular stuffing in the toy. If allergic symptoms develop—watery eyes, sneezing, etc.—consult your physician.

Toys of many kinds become more important as the child grows. As he plays, he learns. Keep in mind the capacities of your child. For the age group under one year, avoid take-apart and noise-making items. Read labels for recommended ages. Assume the toy will end up in the mouth or being chewed: buy items which are labeled "non-toxic." Examine all toys often. Repair damaged toys when possible so they will be safe again, and throw away those that cannot be mended.

Remember not to be caught up by fads in toys: buy what is safe and useful. The most common mistake parents make is buying costly and meaningless playthings for which their children are not ready. This is true for all age groups and will be discussed again in later sections. Use instead pots, pans, and *large* spoons which have no sharp edges. Make use of other items in the home which are safe for baby, already available for other purposes, and cost you nothing.

Sudden Infant Death

This phenomenon, also called crib or cot death, continues to baffle the medical profession and strikes down some 10,000 or more infants in this country annually during the first year of life. As yet, this syndrome is neither predictable nor preventable. Since the exact cause of crib deaths is unknown, specific preventive measures cannot be firmly recommended. However, there are a few suggestions that may avert such tragedies in the first year of life:

1. Feed the infant while you are in a sitting position. Do not leave him alone in the crib with a bottle.

2. Dress the baby in loose clothes for sleeping and do not put a pillow in the crib.

3. Ventilate the baby's room at frequent intervals.

4. Consult a physician as soon as an infant develops a significant cold or respiratory symptom.

5. Report any episodes of unusual temporary interruption in breathing to your physician.

The sudden and unexpected death of apparently thriving infants represents an appalling tragedy to families of victims. The following national parent groups have local chapters throughout the country which can give much understanding and psychological support when needed:

National Foundation for Sudden Infant
  Death, Inc.
1501 Broadway
New York, New York 10036
Telephone (212) 563-4630

International Guild for Infant Survival
7501 Liberty Road
Baltimore, Maryland 21207
Telephone (301) 944-2502

Safety Summary: From Birth to 12 Months

An infant is dependent on his parents for almost everything—food, clothing, shelter, education—but most of all for love and protection. Your child can have a contented, productive and healthy life; your guidance and protective support will help him to achieve his heritage of health.

Suffocation, falls, poisonings, drownings, and burns cause more deaths in this age group than all diseases combined. Safety habits must begin at birth.

- Never underestimate the rapid rate of a baby's physical, mental and social development.
- Always be prepared for the unexpected.

- Never leave a baby alone outside the crib or playpen when he is awake.
- Never leave a baby alone on anything from which he may fall.
- Never leave a baby alone when he is in the tub.
- Keep all objects and substances out of reach.
- Toys should never be smaller than the baby's mouth.
- Begin using the word "no" only when necessary, and follow through on what you have said. Be consistent.

FROM AGES ONE THROUGH FIVE

4

The major causes of deaths to children due to accidents, from ages one through five, are motor vehicle accidents, burns, falls, and poisoning.

The growth and development of your child during these years are exciting and challenging. He has ideas of his own and is increasing his capacity to carry out these ideas. His captive days of crib, infant seat, or playpen will diminish and finally disappear, to make way for explorations of himself and all that is around him.

Recognize that, as your child grows physically, he changes socially as well. Within each stage of growth and development there will be transition periods during which your child must learn to move about in different environments and react to a greater variety of people. You should be aware of the need to train your child in safety techniques, just as you help him learn table manners, how to use toilet facilities, and dress himself.

The average one-year-old child pulls himself to his feet, walks with help, creeps or hitches along, and cooperates while being dressed. He holds a cup to drink, uses a spoon, plays with blocks, but is not yet able to be constructive.

By fifteen months, he can walk alone, stoops to recover toys on the floor, rolls or tosses a ball back to someone, and drinks from a cup without spilling much.

At eighteen months, the average child walks alone well, climbs down the stairs, uses a spoon without much spilling, and shows dramatic imitation in play. From this time

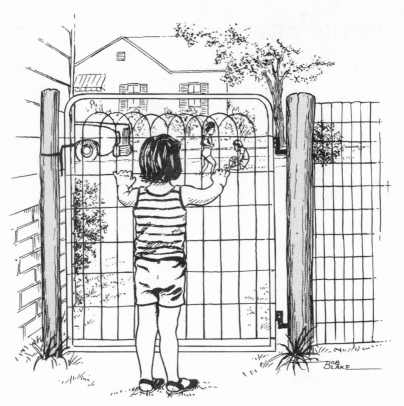

Be prepared for your child's explorations of the world outside.

on to his third birthday, your child is constantly developing and improving his physical skills: he begins to run better and faster, kicks a ball, holds a glass with one hand, and can learn simple physical movements, such as jumping, skipping, and dancing to a favorite melody.

This is the time when you must determine what approach to teach safety habits is best and most comfortable for your child and for you, and in tune with your life style, or family pattern. You must begin to talk with your child about what it is you are doing to protect him and you must enlist his help to prevent accidents.

Your two-year-old probably knows approximately 300 words, makes two-word sentences. He runs, kicks a ball, builds a tower of four to six blocks, holds a glass with one hand, hunts for missing toys, turns pages one at a time, distinguishes between "mine" and "yours." He pouts, dawdles, executes simple commands, imitates simple movements, repeats words, and selects a bright-colored object placed among dull-colored ones of the same size and shape.

However, the toddler's mobility brings with it an age of accidents. The toddler moves quickly but has little appreciation of impending danger. As his curiosity grows, your job will involve more supervision as well as education. At this age the child is learning obedience, which often must be absolute. At the toddler age, children must be protected and *taught by action, as well as words*. This is tiring and difficult for parents, but a child must be removed from danger again and again, with the action supplemented by simple words such as "no."

Doors which lead to stairways, driveways, and storage areas should be securely fastened. Gates across stairways (top and bottom), guards at upstairs windows and hooks high up on doors are helpful in preventing falls. Make sure that the screens in your windows are sturdy and well fastened and cannot be pushed out, especially in the baby's room. Make a practice of opening windows from the top only.

At about three years of age, your child will like to solve ball and box puzzles, turn sharp corners while running, pedal a tricycle; can jump in place, and wash and dry his hands. A child of four can broad-jump, throw a ball overhand, button his clothes, and play together with other children in games like tag. The five-year-old can hop two or more times, catch a ball, and dress and undress himself.

The child's world expands rapidly, and the danger of accidents increases. He isn't content with just his own backyard; he ventures out into the neighborhood, begins

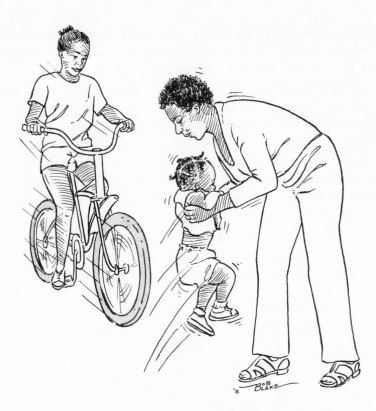

A child must be removed from danger again and again, with the action supplemented by simple words such as "no."

to have playmates, climbs, rides tricycles and plays rough games. He asks "why" to everything. The time has come for more intensive instruction in safety. He must understand the role he has in protecting himself; you must continue to instruct and encourage him in developing self-discipline appropriate to his age and activities.

Children at this stage begin to identify with specific adults. They want to be like a grown-up they love. While there are occasional rebellions, they are generally cooperative about following directions. At the same time, this is a period of intense curiosity and vivid imagination. Attention to safety in this stage must take into account these social and emotional factors in combination with changing physical skills. Teach him by words, but always reinforce your lesson by your own good example.

Teach toddlers the meaning of "hot." Say "HOT!" if you see a youngster about to touch a hot pan or a lighted cigarette. Teach children to stay away from stoves, open fires, hot liquids on stoves, lighters and matches. Place highchairs away from the stove, and turn pot handles toward the back, not the front, of the stove. Keep dishes and containers of hot food and liquids in the center of the table, out of the child's reach.

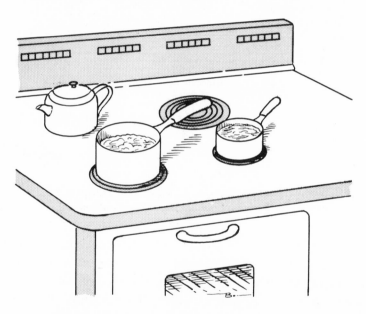

Turn pot handles toward the back, not the front, of the stove.

Play Areas

Fence the child's play yard. *Never* leave small children alone in the house! *Never* leave a small child unattended in a baby carriage or in an automobile. Keep your child away from the street and driveway. Remember that accidents are more frequent when playmates are older. The two-year-old may be easily hurt by bats, hard balls, bicycles, and rough play. Check his play area for hazards that attract attention, such as old refrigerators, deep holes, construction sites, trash heaps, rickety play houses or doghouses, and abandoned buildings. Check on his activities frequently.

Water Hazards and Safety

Most children love the water and should be allowed to enjoy its pleasures, but *with adult supervision*. Drownings happen more often at or near home than at a beach or public pool, and one-third of the victims are one year old or under. Treacherous waters include backyard pools, shallow ponds, brooks, creeks, wells, cisterns, rivers, and lakes. Water is not safe until a child learns to respect it, probably not sooner than four or five years of age. *Never* leave your child without adult supervision in the tub or wading pool, or around open or frozen bodies of water, including yours or your neighbor's swimming pool. Even shallow water is dangerous for the unattended child. Water accidents are second only to motor vehicle ones.

Your home bathtub can be the ideal place to introduce your baby to water exercises that will help him be better prepared for next summer and all the other summers in his life. Especially for babies under one year of age, the use of the tub is very beneficial and enjoyable.

Since your baby has lived in the fluid world of the mother's womb for nine months, he will naturally be comfortable in water if he is introduced to it very early. This natural ease in water is quite a contrast to the common sight of older children clinging to their mothers because of water fear.

Teaching your baby to be happy and confident in water helps both of you in many ways. Most importantly, it can make him "water safe" very early. He learns to enjoy water instead of fear it. And teaching him things in the water gives you and your baby one more way to learn, play, and discover together.

Here's how to begin to teach your baby to swim in your own bathtub. Fill your bath with as much clean, clear water as possible so that it will not overflow when you get in the bathtub. Pick a time when you have 20-30 minutes to work with him. Following are some bathtub exercises, beginning with the simplest and progressing to the more difficult. (If you have any doubts about doing these exercises with your baby, check with your physician.)

A beginning exercise for you and your baby in the tub is bubble blowing. This is an important exercise that should be done daily for several minutes. Hold your baby facing you with your fingers toward his back and pointing upward to his head and neck for support. Your thumbs should be under and around his arms. Hold his head level with yours so that he can see your face. Take a small breath. Gently blow a little air in your baby's face. Continue to blow and then lower your mouth into the water. Keep your neck straight while you blow so that your baby can see the bubbles. *Keep the baby's head above water.* You will have to do this exercise over and over again for your baby. He will learn to blow bubbles on his own simply by imitating.

Probably the most important thing you can accomplish with bathtub exercises is back floating. Your baby will learn this more easily and quickly if you begin at an early age. Before he is eight months old, the bath is usually adequate for floating. After eight months, if he is not already floating, he will be able to touch the sides of the tub.

To hold your baby for the back floating position (with

you out of the tub), support him with one hand under his neck and one hand on the leg nearest you. Gently move him backward and forward along the surface of the water. Don't let any water splash on his face, but do hold him low enough to cover his ears with water.

Practice back floating with your baby at least 10 minutes a day. If you are patient and regular in your practice of the back float, your baby may be able to float alone by the time he can hold his head steady (between 3 and 5 months).

You can also help your baby practice back floating while you are in the tub with him. Sit with your legs apart. Hold your baby with his head away from your body. Your hands should be on each side of his back, with your thumbs under and around his arms toward the chest. If your baby is not yet able to hold his head securely on his own, be sure to extend your fingers to provide head support. When you feel your baby is relaxed enough to float alone, gradually release your grip. Stay close to him so that you can quickly give support if he needs it. With regular practice, babies can turn themselves onto their backs to float by the time they are eight to nine months old.*

Start swimming instructions early (about age three). Teach your child the water-survival technique as described and illustrated on pp. 106-107.

Teach your children basic swimming safety rules:

- Swim only in supervised areas, and never dive into strange waters or into shallow breaking waves at the beach.
- Stay out of the water during storms, particularly if there is lightning!

* For other and more detailed bathtub water exercises read *How to Teach Your Baby to Swim* by Claire Timmermans, published in 1975 by Stein and Day, New York.

- At a pool, do not allow running, pushing, or dunking in or near the pool.
- Keep glasses and bottles away from the pool.
- In lakes and ponds, avoid swimming in areas immediately in front of steep, sloping banks.
- Do not swim in areas where there are motor boats and fishing lines.
- Don't yell "help" unless you mean it (remember the boy who repeatedly cried "wolf"!).

Preventing Suffocation

Children should not be allowed to eat while walking or running around. Nuts, popcorn, hard candy, and so forth should be kept away from children until the age of at least four years, and then only when they are seated and quiet. The habit of putting pins, coins, and similar objects in the mouth should be prevented by direction and parental example.

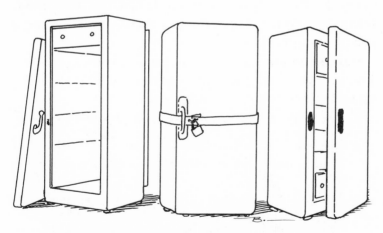

Discarded refrigerators can be rendered harmless by removing the door; locking the door so that it cannot open; drilling holes in the cabinet and removing the latch and handle; or having the refrigerator removed to a junkyard and destroyed.

All too frequently one reads of a child suffocating from entrapment in a refrigerator, an entirely preventable accident. Discarded refrigerators, freezers, small ice chests, and airtight containers are inviting places for games by small children. All too often they result in needless deaths. All of these death traps can be rendered harmless by removing the door or the latch stop so that the door cannot close or lock; drilling holes in the cabinet and removing the gasket; or better by destroying the box altogether or having it carted away.

Tell your child it is absolutely forbidden to push another child into such an enclosure, and if he sees another child push a playmate into a refrigerator, or similar appliance he should help him out immediately, if he can, but waste no time in reporting the situation to an adult. Explain to your child the dangers a discarded refrigerator or freezer holds—he may not be able to get out without help and no one will hear him if he cries; he cannot be seen; and he may not be able to breathe.

Poisoning

Poisonous substances are discussed in detail in Chapter 6. Here only some general guidelines are offered.

Fatal poisonings are most frequent between the ages of one and three. Children often explore with taste, and a child should be allowed to taste something unpleasant such as a minimal amount of vinegar or mustard with the warning that he will not like it. Soon he will learn that not everything is pleasant to eat.

It is of particular importance to teach your child in ways which will help him develop self-control. He will find himself in situations which offer more opportunity for access to poisons, and he must begin to learn to discriminate and to protect himself outside of the home.

Simple, inexpensive, easily installed safety latches (Kindergard™) are available for cabinets and drawers containing medicines, drugs, or poisonous household agents. Use them to insure protection for your child.

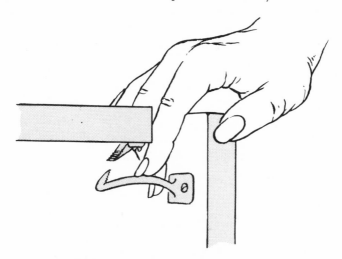

Simple, inexpensive, easily installed safety latches (Kindergard™) are available for cabinets and drawers.

Toys

Toys are more than mere amusing devices. The child achieves and grows by play; toys are his tools. Children from the ages of one to three especially like toys to push and pull, such as simple wooden and plastic toys on wheels and push-pull tops. They also will enjoy large peg boards; large, smooth building blocks with rounded corners; a sand box with sturdy rust-proof pail and shovel; colorful picture books; cuddly toys for naptime; play-size tables and chairs without sharp edges; rubber or plastic balls; and sturdy cars and wagons.

It is essential that children be given safe toys which they can be taught to use properly. Guides to help parents keep unsafe toys away from children include: (1) The Good Housekeeping Consumers Guaranty Seal, which *Good Housekeeping* magazine allows manufacturers who advertise in their magazine to put on toys it has investigated and accepted for performance and safety; (2) the *Underwriters' Laboratories, Inc.* label (UL), the standard of safety for everything electrical; (3) "no-advertising" magazines which maintain testing laboratories and publish reports on such items as electric trains, slot cars, and tricycles; (4) the *American Academy of Pediatrics' Accident Prevention Committee*, which acts as a toy safety clearinghouse, reports on hazardous toys and calls them to the attention of the public and the *National Safety Council*; (5) the *Safety Standards Committee of the Toy Manufacturers of the Toy Manufacturers of the U.S.A., Inc.*, which has been studying and recommending safety standards for toys

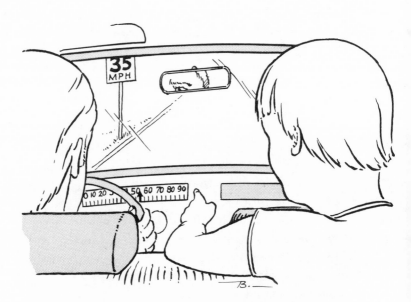

Your child must be taught by what you say, but what you say must be reinforced by your own example.

since 1955; and (6) the *United States Consumers Product Safety Commission*.

Summary: Ages One Through Five

A child of one through five lives in the age of accidents. The child learns to sit, crawl, stand, and walk. His curiosity is full-blown. His world is expanding rapidly as he ventures "out" into an ever-widening environment. He can be quite cooperative and, even while asking "why" to everything, is eager to imitate the adults he loves. The time has come for more intensive instruction in safety.

He must be taught by what you tell him, but this must be reinforced by your own example. He observes how you cross the street, sees you work with tools or in the kitchen, is aware of how you drive your car. His belief in what you say as demonstrated by what you do is very important in giving him a good educational base for his future well-being.

FROM AGES SIX THROUGH FOURTEEN

5

The major causes of injury and death due to accidents for children of ages six through fourteen involve motor vehicles, fires, burns, falls, and drownings.

These years are ones of great change in the child and adaptation on the part of the adult who is responsible for his care. These are the years during which your child develops his own individuality. Babyhood and toddler adventures are past, but the responsibilities and satisfactions of adulthood are still in the distant future. Your child, with loving protection from you, increases his freedom and expands his ability to take care of himself.

Your child is developing skills, trying new ideas, considering what he wants for himself. He needs to be allowed to make decisions, be successful, make mistakes, and try again.

Parents have to understand their child's increasingly independent behavior. Guidance must be firm but not stifling. Encouragement and persuasion become more important than absolute protection and obedience.

These are the years during which your child develops physical power through body growth and development. Before he can trust himself to use that power he begins to realize that he must earn the respect of other people by considering them, too. He learns the more mature meanings of sharing, self-control, obedience. He needs opportunities to develop these traits.

The Urge To Explore

It is characteristic of a child during these years to explore vigorously through unending play. As your child matures, play and daily living increasingly involve reality: having a real wrist watch; helping cook a meal; using adult-size tools for real jobs around the home. Play changes from exploration and experimentation to the use of developing skills in attempts to accomplish more complex and responsible tasks: riding a bike as a means of transportation to school; having a newspaper route; doing yard work.

Your child's individuality is important to him, but at the same time he still wants and needs rules to live by. These rules take on new meaning, changing from the younger child's simplistic view that a rule must never be broken to the older child's understanding that rules are related to principles upon which a civilized society is based. As his awareness of these principles improves he is developing a greater capacity for self-control and self-discipline and an awareness of his part in the world around him.

Self-control and Self-discipline

Your child's capacity to protect himself from accidents during these ages is directly related to his development of self-control, self-discipline, and understanding of his own role in taking care of himself. It becomes less likely as well as less desirable to protect your child from exposure to all possible hazards. It is more worth while to improve your child's ability to handle dangerous situations than to restrict necessary and desirable behavior, so important for his on-going growth and development. Parents should understand that once a child in this age range is exposed to danger, he often has some control over possible injury by the way he reacts. He will make decisions, some with deliberate effort and some quite automatically, which will either reduce or make him prone to the risk of injury.

At about the age of six, most children become daily travelers to and from school. Whether they are pedestrians, bike riders, or are transported in buses or cars, all need specific information about how to carry out this daily routine safely.

As pedestrians, children are often injured because of darting into the road or street. Teach your child to use crosswalks, walk on sidewalks where available, or walk on the left side of the road facing traffic. Tell him to be cautious even at stop signs, changing traffic lights, or at crosswalks. Being "right" doesn't help the tragedy of an accident.

Defensive Behavior

Your child is beginning to learn *defensive behavior:* he must understand that while rules are to be followed he must expect that others may not follow these rules all the time. He has to be prepared to anticipate the wrong actions of others.

When your child rides a bike to school, he must understand the basic rules of stopping at intersections, signalling for turns, and knowing the right of way. But again, be sure that your child is old enough or capable enough to cope safely with the complexities of in-traffic bike riding. *Most first graders are not.* The seemingly simple task of using one arm to indicate the desire to make a turn will cause many six-year-olds to lose control of steering.

Children who are transported to and from school in buses and cars must learn how to get in and out of the vehicles safely and to avoid carelessly stepping out into traffic. They must learn to behave properly in the vehicle so that excessive noise and horseplay do not distract the driver.

Teaching your child safety habits also gives him a sense of your love and concern. Together you are talking about his own sense of worth, enlisting his help to continue caring for himself.

Summary: Ages Six Through Fourteen

These patterns of learning rules, using self-control, and behaving defensively must be continued throughout this growth period in preparation for the greater independence of the years which follow. Protection from

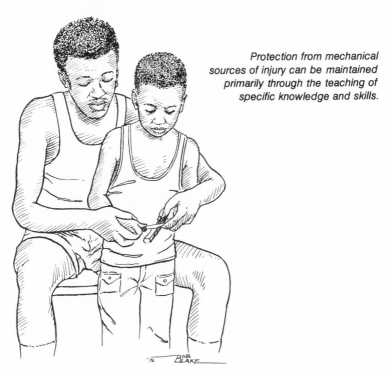

Protection from mechanical sources of injury can be maintained primarily through the teaching of specific knowledge and skills.

mechanical sources of injury can be maintained primarily through the teaching of specific knowledge and skills. Protection from emotional challenges which may interfere with comfortable maturation and safety can be maintained through the interaction of the child with the people who love and care for him. He will generally be contented and cooperative when he is satisfied with himself and with what is happening around him. You must be alert to stresses which result in his confusion, self-doubt, poor school performance, and judgment.

Late in this stage of growth some of the most serious challenges to a child's safety will involve emotion-based reactions to demands and ideas of the child's peers, or playmates. Drugs, alcohol, sex, and automobiles become tantalizing temptations. You need to know the facts about the dangers as well as the kinds of pressure the child may be experiencing to participate in forbidden activities. Some of these activities occasionally are the "in thing to do" for the child and hard to resist. You must continue to reinforce the earlier habits of self-control and independent judgment that the child needs and can exercise.

A less well-recognized source of danger is that of the runaway child. Authorities estimate that there are more than one million runaways each year and of these approximately *one third are fourteeen years old or younger*. Information about children who run away shows that they do so for a variety of reasons and situations:

- Divorce, alcoholism, or illness of parents
- Constant family hassles about such things as "long hair," dress, and personal appearance
- Parents who appear to the child to be demoralized by unfulfilling work and private life

Whether the child is right or wrong, his perception of events around him and in which he must play a part causes him to act in certain ways. You need to review your family situation and take constructive action when there are excessive tensions and problems. Sometimes directly dealing with these problems with all family members present can be successful. Community sources should be used when necessary. These resources include personal physicians, community mental health centers, alcoholics and gamblers anonymous centers, family service agencies, ministers, and a variety of other individuals and organizations trained to help us all through times of severe stress.

Your response to "emotional hazards" is really not very different from that needed for "mechanical hazards." Protection, discipline, regulation, and teaching are the intervention choices that can be used.

Handicapped Children: Safe Independence

Children who are handicapped require the same attention to safety that other children do: attention which changes as growth and development stages change and which provides opportunities for trial, error, and success in controlled settings before going out on their own. In addition, handicapped children may require *modifications in living arrangements and equipment which will enhance growth towards self-control, self-protection, and independence*.

We cannot do more here than touch on some of the functional areas that coincide with the needs of handicapped children throughout their growth and development. Parents of handicapped children should make the fullest use of specific resources available to them, whether for understanding their child's handicap, for ideas about making home life more comfortable, or enabling free entry of the child into all aspects of society.

We suggest you consider the special safety needs of your handicapped child by asking yourself the following questions:

1. In what way does this handicap require me to do something extra or different to help him avoid hazards?

2. How can I provide any needed special help most simply, using short cuts and adapting what is at hand?

Any modifications made in the home should enhance the handicapped child's ability and potential to learn to take care of himself in ways appropriate to his age and also make it easier to provide necessary care for the child. As an example, for the child who has a physical handicap that interferes with walking or requires the use of crutches, braces, or a wheel chair, you would need to focus attention on some specific areas of the home:

1. Bathrooms: non-skid tub and floors; railings in the tub.
2. All floors: non-skid surfaces; carpeting fastened firmly; door sills eliminated or modified.
3. Furniture placement: to minimize tripping; to allow easy use with special equipment such as crutches.
4. Stairways: railings on both sides; good lighting; change to ramp with railings if possible.

Evacuation procedures in the event of fire should be given extra attention. Special help is generally available through local fire departments. Inspections of the home will be made by fire department personnel so they are fully informed about the best ways of removing the handicapped person from *your particular setting*. They will also provide special luminous decals which are generally placed in two locations (see illustration): on the window of the room in which the handicapped person spends a lot of time or sleeps; on the front door so that it is immediately visible from the street in the event of fire. This symbol is used throughout the United States. In communities where such a program does not exist, it can probably be developed on request and is not expensive to the community. Where the program does exist, it is funded either through civic groups or tax revenues: there is no cost to the handicapped.

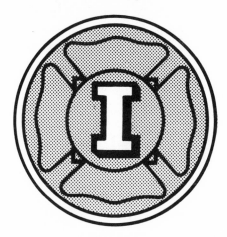

Fire Department personnel will provide special luminous decals where there are handicapped children in a home.

If your child was born with a handicap, chances are that you were soon offered names of people and organizations you could turn to for assistance. If a handicap is a result of disease or injury (which is the more frequent way children become handicapped), your physician or other sources of care during the illness or after the injury probably suggested sources of continuing help for rehabilitation. But sometimes this information is not sufficient for a variety of reasons: all of the demands placed on parents whose children do not have handicaps are intensified for those parents whose children are handicapped.

Identify one or more resources who offer not only specific help such as rehabilitation care, speech therapy, or medical care, but also can be used by you for periodic review to see where you are, how things seem to you. It will continue to be important to talk throughout your child's growth and development with persons experienced in providing help and information to the handicapped.

In addition to using your physician, you may wish to obtain information and help from many sources that are available in your community for the handicapped individual such as:

- Health department
- Medical school
- Diagnostic treatment or rehabilitation centers
- Local chapters of national health organizations which serve the handicapped

PART THREE

Hazards

INTRODUCTION

In previous chapters we discussed stages of child growth and development as they relate to the safety of your child. Now, we focus on specific hazards, in the hope that we can help you avoid such hazards or encounter them less often.

Accidents occur most often when your child cannot react safely because the threat of the situation is beyond his capacity to cope with it, whether because of specific behavior or product use. You must be able to recognize at what age a particular situation or product use is dangerous for a child. For example, a ten-year-old child lacks the necessary physical, social, and emotional development to drive a car safely. Many less obvious situations are equally dangerous.

Learn the characteristics of a product that may be handled or used by your child. Anticipate the dangers of a situation in which your child may find himself. We are using the term "product" to include a multitude of items encountered daily by any child, including medicines, fabrics, tools, electrical sources, appliances, motor vehicles, farm machinery, swimming pools, toys, household goods, chemicals (insectides, etc.), building materials.

In considering products *to which children up to the age of 14 are likely to be exposed*, three general product characteristics must be kept in mind:

1. Products highly dangerous and likely to cause injury—for example, guns, poisons, and fireworks.

2. Products less likely to lead to injury except when used in an unusual or unintended way—for example, plastic bags, discarded refrigerators.

3. Products less likely to lead to accidents but, more importantly, can be expected to cause severe and sudden injury—for example, glass doors and windows of non-safety glass, flammable fabrics, lawn mowers, motor vehicle use without restraints.

You must consider, then, whether the use or safe exposure to a given product will require:

- No specific experience or training
- A little or a lot of physical strength
- No judgment or sophisticated judgment

Consideration of these potentials of your child will enable you to decide when your child can be exposed to or use safely a particular product or carry out a particular task.

A "safe" environment, such as your home, is not without hazards. Nor does a safe living pattern mean constant restrictions, shouts of warnings, or nagging cautions. A safe living pattern is one in which your child learns to anticipate hazards which have been reduced to a minimum and, through knowledge and habits of self-control, can cope with those hazards, even if they occur in unaccustomed or new situations. The following chapters offer specific information about common hazards.

POISONING: A COMMON EMERGENCY

6

General Precautions

Poisoning is the most common *medical* emergency among young children. The curiosity of children tempts them to sample the thousands of products, many with potentially poisonous chemicals, and the myriad of prescribed and over-the-counter medicines or drugs—many of which are often present in your home.

Prevention of poisoning accidents must be based on a philosophy of "out of sight, out of reach and locked away." This is because the age group most frequently involved in poisoning accidents is under five years of age. It is more practical to change the physical environment in which your toddler moves about than to try to maintain the strict control that otherwise would be necessary. Of all poisonings in children under five years of age, 75 percent are caused by *in sight* drugs or household cleaning agents. Three out of four of these tragic events could have been prevented by just *one* very simple action—putting all drugs and household cleaning agents *out of sight* and *out of reach* of these children.

However, your children remain in continuous danger because you cannot constantly supervise all of their activities, especially when they may be visiting elsewhere. Therefore, your efforts to help your child develop *self-control* and *disinterest* in these poisonous substances are essential.

You, no doubt, seldom have deliberately gone shop-

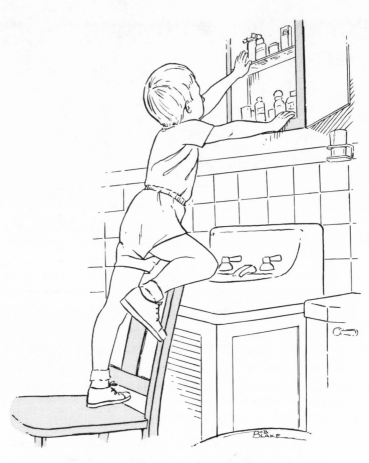

Store all medicines and drugs out of sight and reach, preferably in a locked cabinet.

ping for poisons, but the fact is that you buy several every time you go to the grocery, hardware, or drugstore. Poisons are in many products which you use every day. It may be difficult for you to believe that your child will swallow horrible-tasting things like dishwasher detergent, bleach, furniture polish, and drain cleaners. But your child of age five years or less explores his world with hand and mouth. This hand-to-mouth behavior is quite normal and frequent up to the age of about two, but can continue intermittently for several years beyond. Your child will explore and experiment and taste before discovering he does not like it. Tragically, *one taste* can lead to severe poisoning.

Accept the fact that your child will explore, that he has the capacity to open containers of all kinds, and that he cares little or nothing about how it tastes. Precautions must be taken and safe habits practiced.

Chemical Hazards

Medicines and Drugs

- Store all medicines and drugs *out of sight and reach*, preferably in a locked cabinet, separate from food.
- Safety caps are now required by law for many drugs and household cleaning agents. Purchase products with safety caps or in safety containers.
- Always read labels before using any medicine or drug. Do not reuse the container for any other product.
- The name of the drug should appear on all prescription labels for rapid identification.
- Containers of similar size, shape, and labeling should not be placed next to each other in the medicine cabinet.
- Never allow anyone else, even an older child, to get medicine for you.
- Clean out medicine cabinets periodically (at least twice a year), and dispose of old medicines by flushing them down the drain. Rinse out empty containers before putting them in the trash.
- Prescription medicines should be discarded when the illness for which they were prescribed has run its course.

- Don't give medicines prescribed for one child to another child. Let your physician advise which drugs are safe for all children, such as cough syrup.
- Never give or take medicines in the dark.

Medicines should be regarded by children seriously and with a matter-of-fact attitude. Don't make it a big production. Giving medicine should not be made a game. Drugs should never be referred to as "candy," and children should never be bribed by such inducements. They should be taught to respect medicines as an aid to regaining good health when sick.

Your attitudes and behavior can influence your children's attitudes toward medicine, perhaps for the rest of their lives. *Do not deceive your children about medicines*; tell them the truth.

Household Cleaning Agents and Garden Supplies

Store out of sight and reach, preferably in a locked cabinet, separate from food. Always read the label and use only as directed.

After use, do not leave household and garden supplies open or within reach of children. If you have to leave the room, even for an instant, cap all products such as furniture polish, insecticides, or drain cleaners, and place them in a location inaccessible to your child.

Keep all household and garden supplies in their *original containers with labels intact*. A tragic number of accidents happen because poisonous materials are placed in soda pop bottles, cider jugs, cereal or candy boxes, milk cartons, cake tins, coffee cans, cups, and other containers which children associate with food and drink. Kerosene stored in tin cans, glass jugs, or coke bottles has resulted in many accidental poisonings, as has charcoal grill lighter fluid kept in a soft drink bottle.

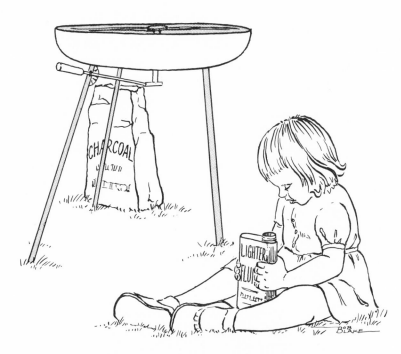

Do not leave outdoor grill and garden supplies containing poisons open or within reach of children.

Be sure that container caps are tight and containers are intact. Leaking containers and their content should be disposed of immediately. Better waste the contents than try to save them in another container. Dispose of containers following approved local procedures in order to avoid contaminating water supplies or causing danger to other people.

Pesticides which have come under government restrictions should be stored out of reach and sight until facilities for their disposal are set up by your community.

To prevent re-use of empty poison containers, carefully mutilate (puncture plastic containers) and crush completely. Then wrap the empty, rinsed, and destroyed containers in several thick layers of newspaper, tie securely, and place in the trash cans for disposal.

Aerosol Containers

- Read the label and use only as directed.
- Always have adequate ventilation when using.
- Remember that not only the toxic product (such as an insecticide) but also the propellent is hazardous. (Trying to get "high" from sniffing freon propellents has produced a number of deaths in teenagers. The use of freon gas as a propellent is being phased out in this country, because of the controversy over its effect on the ozone layer of the atmosphere.)
- Never puncture or burn aerosol containers. Do not expose them to heat. The container can explode, releasing harmful chemical fumes.
- Dispose of aerosol containers by wrapping in newspaper, tie the package, and place in covered trash cans inaccessible to children. If there is another prescribed method recommended in your community, use it.

Summary of Poisonous Products

There are many attractively packaged and enticing household products available for children to experiment with and taste. The following outline offers general groupings by potential poisoning level related to the amount found in a particular item. For example, if a child bites a flashlight battery he may swallow ingredients that are defined as poisons, but are relatively harmless in the amounts present in flashlight batteries.

Extremely harmful *(ingestion requires urgent medical care)*

Cleaning, polishing and bleaching products
Detergents for laundry and dishwashers
Metal cleaners and polishes

Ammonia, bleach, and dry-cleaning fluid
Polishes and waxes for furniture, floors, shoes
Paints, paint removers, varnishes
Kerosene, gasoline, lighter fluids
Hair preparations including shampoos and rinse items for streaking, coloring, rinsing, and tinting
Roach tablets and powders; ant poisons; rat poisons; and other strong insecticides and pesticides.

Moderately harmful *(no medical treatment is required unless large quantities are ingested)*

After-shave lotion	Fish bowl agents
Cosmetics	Pencil lead
Flashlight batteries	Play-dough
Bubble bath	Shaving cream
Candles	Bar soap
Deodorizer cakes	Mercury (from broken
Caps for toy pistols	thermometer)
Most house plants	Tooth paste

Carbon Monoxide

Carbon monoxide is a colorless, odorless, and poisonous gas. It can cause illness and death as it accumulates in any confined area. Most people know that leaving a car engine running in a garage is unsafe not only for those in the garage but also for persons in the attached living areas. Carbon monoxide can penetrate through any opening.

Other sources of carbon monoxide leakage—and thus danger—are any fuel-burning apparatus such as gas space heaters, stoves, furnaces. Such equipment should comply with all local codes and carry a national testing agency seal indicating that it meets with national safety standards. Proper installation and maintenance are essential.

Adequate ventilation in campers, tents, and trailers is also necessary. Automobile station wagon tailgate windows, when open, will pull in carbon monoxide: always open other windows to produce a safe air flow.

Burning charcoal in grills and hibachis is also a source of carbon monoxide gas. Never use them in enclosed areas, without adequate ventilation.

Lead Poisoning

In the home the main source of lead poisoning is dried, peeling paint on walls, woodwork, repainted furniture, and painted toys. Children suck and chew on toys and furniture all the time. They will pick at peeling paint and loose plaster until they pull off a piece or find flakes which fall on the floor—and into the mouth it goes. If you repaint anything inside or outside your house, use only unaltered lead-free paint.

Even if you do paint with lead-free paint, there may be layers of old paint underneath that have a high lead content. Take no chances: scrape off *all* the layers of old or peeling paint. Wrap the scrapings in newspapers or bags, tie securely, and dispose in a covered garbage container out of sight and reach of children.

Be sure that your floors are always clean—never leave bits and pieces of flaked paint on them.

When your child is outdoors, however, you will have to keep a watchful eye. Many outdoor paints—especially on windows—flake off easily. Teach your child not to chew or eat any flakes on window sills, putty, porch steps, iron gates, and trellises. Color-tinted newspapers and ceramic glaze also have a high content of lead.

Some infants display an "unusual" appetite for inedible substances such as paint chips, plaster, crayons, chalk, wallpaper, newspaper (especially if tinted), dirt, and cigarettes. This abnormal craving is called "pica." A child with this tendency must be well-protected; persistent pica can cause lead or other poisoning. If your child shows these symptoms, discuss the problem with your physician.

Food Poisoning

There are four common causes of food poisoning—*Salmonella*, *Clostridium perfringens*, *Staphylococcus*, and *Clostridium botulinum*. These are simple, little bacteria organisms—one-celled organisms that multiply by dividing. To divide they need food, warmth, and moisture. These bacteria may be present in all foods because they are everywhere in the environment. It's up to you to protect yourself and your family from them.

The "infamous four" can cause illness or, in extreme cases, even death.

Many people from the farmer through the retailer work to protect you from these bacteria. The U.S. Department of Agriculture or a state agency inspects your meat and poultry for wholesomeness. The Food and Drug Administration inspects processing plants where all other foods are produced.

But, from the supermarket shelf to the dinner table you are the one responsible for protecting your food. Your responsibility begins in the supermarket. Don't buy any food in containers—cans or packages—that are outdated, broken, bent, or leaky. Especially avoid bulging cans—the food could contain lethal botulism toxin. Let the store manager know there is something wrong so that he can take the package or can off the shelf.

Another thing you can do in the supermarket is to make sure meat, poultry, and frozen foods are kept cold. Buy them last so they don't warm up or defrost in the cart while shopping.

Make the grocery store your last stop so you can go right home. On arriving home, immediately put your meat and poultry in the refrigerator, which should be at 40 degrees F., or in the freezer at 0 degrees F. Put frozen foods in the freezer right away. This prevents any bacteria in the food from growing.

When you take your fresh meat, poultry, or frozen foods out to cook, don't do any favors for the "infamous four." Thaw foods in the refrigerator, or cook them frozen. If you must thaw in a hurry, do so in a water-tight plastic bag submerged in cold water.

Never thaw frozen food uncovered on a kitchen counter at room temperature. Remember, there are bacteria everywhere, and room temperature lets them grow.

The way the "infamous four" usually strikes in the home is through cross-contamination. Since the bacteria are killed under proper cooking temperatures, an illness from cross-contamination can occur only if you've failed to take the right precautions. Here's how that can happen:

Your chicken has been thawed and you have cut it up on your cutting board. You put the chicken into the frying pan and begin preparing your other foods. If you use the same knife and cutting board without first washing them and your hands in soap and hot water, you could contaminate whatever else you prepare.

For example, say you have cooked potatoes for potato salad. You slice them with the same knife on the same cutting board you used for the raw chicken without washing either the board, the knife, or your hands. You could easily spread *Salmonella* bacteria to the potatoes. If you take the salad on a picnic where temperatures are warm enough for bacterial growth, they will multiply rapidly to the levels where infection can occur.

Good habits in the kitchen can help prevent food contamination. For example, don't keep main dishes at room temperature for longer than two hours before serving. Bacteria grow rapidly at room temperature.

Follow simple hygienic practices. Use rubber gloves if you have cuts or sores on your hands. That not only keeps bacteria out of the sores, it also keeps bacteria from the sores from getting on the food.

Put leftovers into the refrigerator as soon as the meal is over. Refrigerate them in small or shallow containers so they will cool quickly.

Pets also are carriers of the "infamous four" bacteria. After handling pets, wash your hands before working with food. Don't allow pet feeding dishes, toys, or bedding in the kitchen. Don't let pets touch food, utensils, or food-working surfaces.

Here are some details about the "infamous four":

Salmonella is one of the most common causes of food poisoning. While it is not often fatal, it is widespread. More than two million cases of illness from *Salmonella* poisoning are believed to occur in the United States each year.

Salmonella is most commonly found in raw meats, poultry, eggs, milk, fish, and products made from them. Other sources can be pets, such as dogs, cats, turtles, birds, and fish.

There is no way to tell by looking at, tasting, or smelling the food whether *Salmonella* germs are present. To avoid them, however, do not handle the food excessively and keep it below 40 degrees F. or above 140 degrees F.

Salmonella germs in food are destroyed by heat. So, always use a meat thermometer and cook foods thoroughly.

Also, heat leftovers thoroughly. Broth and gravies should be brought to a roiling boil for several minutes when reheating.

Symptoms of *Salmonella* infection are fever, headache, diarrhea, abdominal discomfort, and occasionally vomiting. These appear in 24 hours after eating contaminated food. Most people recover in two to four days. Children under 4, the elderly and people already weakened by disease could become seriously ill.

Clostridium perfringens is widely distributed in nature —in the soil, dust, on food, and in the intestinal tracts of man and other warm-blooded animals. It is more widespread over the earth than any other disease-causing micro-organism.

Disease outbreaks frequently occur when foods are held in large quantities at improper temperatures for several hours. Food poisoning due to these germs are closely associated with restaurants or other large feeding establishments where foods are held for long periods of time on steam tables or other warming devices.

To avoid food poisoning from the germs, meats should be properly cooked, held hot (above 140 degrees F.) and served hot. If you cook meat for later use, cool the meat rapidly in small containers in a refrigerator to 40 degrees F. or below. Thoroughly reheat leftover meats or meat dishes before serving—and bring leftover gravy to a roiling boil before serving. Maintain cold cuts and cold sliced meats below 40 degrees F. and serve them cold.

Large numbers of these bacteria can cause diarrhea and abdominal pain in from four to 22 hours—usually in about 12 hours.

Staphylococcus—known as staph—is quite common. Staph organisms are in respiratory passages and on skin. They usually enter food from a human or an animal.

Staph germs grow in a wide variety of foods—all meats, poultry and egg products, egg, tuna, chicken, potato, or macaroni salads, cream filled pastries, and sandwich fillings. If staph germs are allowed to multiply to high levels, they form a toxin which you *cannot* boil or bake away.

Symptoms of staph food poisoning are diarrhea, vomiting, and abdominal cramps. They appear two to four hours after eating and may bother you for 24 to 48 hours. Staph food poisoning is rarely fatal.

Clostridium botulinum, while rare, is usually fatal. A tiny amount of the toxin poison from botulism germs can kill. Botulism spores are found throughout the environment and are harmless. However, in the proper environment, and when not destroyed by heat, the spores divide and produce poisonous toxins. When your child eats food containing the toxin, he can become ill or die. High heat makes the toxin harmless.

Very few deaths from botulism in commercially canned foods have been reported since 1925. But poisoning from home-canned foods happens more often. About 700 people have died from botulism since 1925 from eating contaminated home-canned products.

Undercooking is the real culprit in home-canning. In general, high acid foods may be canned by boiling; but all other, including meats and poultry, should be canned in pressure cookers at the appropriate level for the required length of time.

Signs of botulism poisoning begin 12 to 36 hours after eating the food. They include double vision, inability to swallow, speech difficulty, and progressive paralysis of the respiratory system.

Medical help must be obtained fast. If botulism is suspected, call your doctor immediately.

Salmonella, *perfringens*, and *Staphylococcus* are invisible and can be detected only by a bacteriological test. Botulism may provide its own clues in canned foods. Bulging cans, an off color, unusal odor, or suspect appearance are the tipoff. If in doubt: **Don't eat it! Don't even taste it!** If it's home-canned, throw it away where no person or animal can get to it. Save any commercially canned product you may suspect and report it to the Food and Drug Administration, or your local public health officials.

The "infamous four" are everywhere, but with proper food handling practices, you can prevent them from causing illness in your home.

Plant Poisoning

Plants are third on the list of the most common substances responsible for human poisoning. More than 160,000 reported human poisoning cases a year occur in the United States. Each year, many thousands of children suffer from poisoning due to plants. While most of them do not suffer symptoms that warrant hospitalization, some are severely, even fatally, poisoned—often by only very small amounts of the offending plant (leaves, berries, flowers, roots, stems, bark).

People tend to think that poisonous plants are found only in rural areas or in forests. Not so. Many poisonous plants are found in suburban plantings (for example, rhododendrons and daffodils) and even inside homes growing in pots (for example, philodendron and hyacinths). Unfortunately, few people realize that among their own shrubbery, flowers, and house plants they may have varieties that can be poisonous to their children.

Impress these rules on your children:

- Never to eat any part of a plant. (Your child can be allowed to eat edible berries, such as strawberries, off a plant but only *with your permission*. Also, even vegetables, if not washed thoroughly, can be harmful.)
- To recognize Western poison oak, poison ivy or sumac and avoid all contact.
- To recognize the plants in your home or yard. (It's fun and educational!) But also to beware of poison-

ing, and allergic reactions, and dermatitis, after you have explained the dangers.

- Not to chew on imported beans or seeds.

On your part:

- Keep plants out of reach of children too young to obey your instructions.
- Seek emergency treatment whenever a child shows symptoms due to chewing or swallowing a poisonous plant.
- Seek medical help when symptoms of allergies or dermatitis appear.
- Not to make teas, brews, or home-made medicines of plants.
- Be ready to identify the plant, or to bring along some evidence of it, when you seek medical help. If you cannot get some of the plant itself, you should save some of the plant particles from the child's stool or vomitus.

As a help in recognizing poisoning caused by chewing or swallowing, or direct contact with poisonous plants, the accompanying Guide has been prepared. It lists the most common dangerous plants and their poisonous parts and gives symptoms for each, as well as a short introduction to the three major problems—allergies, dermatitis, and internal poisoning. The plants are listed by their common names.*

---

*For a comprehensive treatment of poisonous plants, see Hardin and Arena, *Human Poisoning from Native and Cultivated Plants* (Duke University Press, 2nd Edition, copyright 1974). Order from your bookstore.

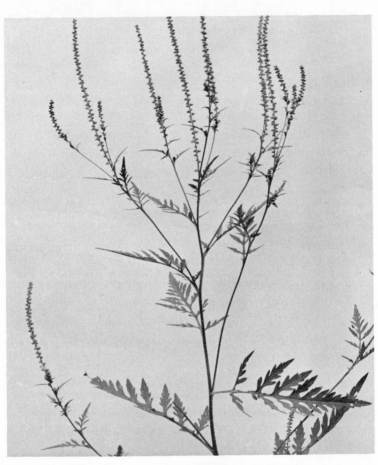

Common ragweed (Ambrosia artemisiifolia). A ubiquitous weed with terminal spikes of numerous pollen flowers.

A Guide to Poisonous Plants

ALLERGIES

Thousands of children suffer from allergies which, if untreated, may lead to asthma and other serious complications. You should see your physician if your child shows signs of allergy—continual sneezing, watery eyes,

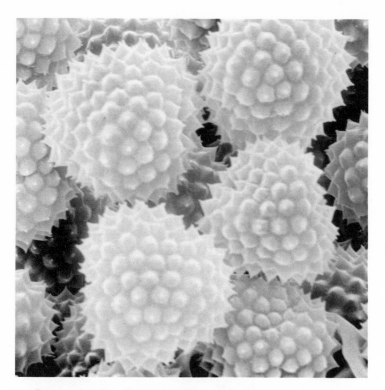

Ragweed pollen (Ambrosia trifida). Scanning electron micrograph; magnification 1,744 times. One grain has a diameter of 20 microns, or 0.02 millimeter, or 0.0007 inch. Courtesy of Dr. W. W. Payne and Ms. Joan M. Courvoisier, Department of Botany, University of Illinois.

stopped-up nose, breathing difficulty persisting over a period of weeks.

Seasonally, early spring brings on pollen from, primarily, deciduous trees such as oak, elm, cedar, maple, sycamore, ash, alder, birch, poplar, beech, and others, all of which may cause allergic symptoms. The problem of treatment is complicated by the great number of trees and shrubs involved.

In midsummer, the allergies are caused primarily by grasses of various types, some herbs, and a few late-flowering trees.

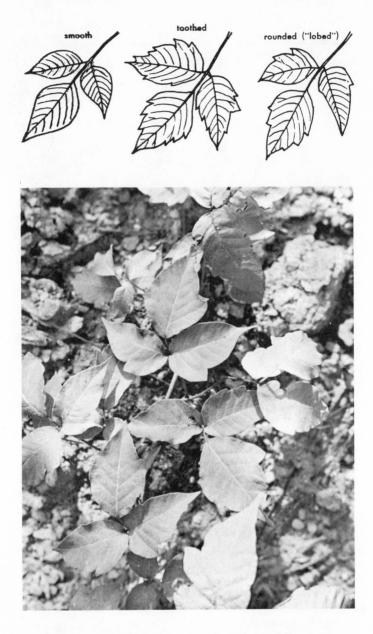

smooth   toothed   rounded ("lobed")

Poison ivy (Toxicodendron radicans). *The infamous weed of the United States and Canada with the characteristic three leaflets. Outlines show variation of the leaflet margin; the lobed form is similar to poison oak. USDA photograph.*

In the fall, ragweed is the most common offender. Common ragweed is illustrated on page 84.

DERMATITIS

Irritation to the skin, or dermatitis, can be caused by numerous plants. It is dependent on the individual child's sensitivity to a particular plant. (Again, consult your physician when the symptoms first occur.)

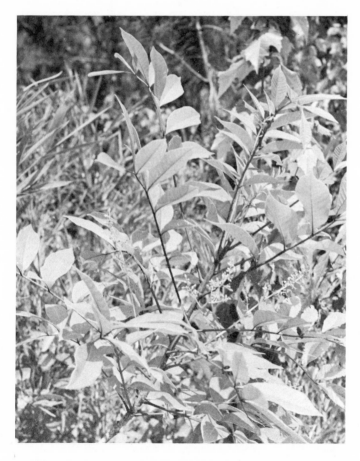

Poison sumac (Toxicodendron vernix). A poisonous shrub of bogs and swamps.

The degree of poisoning may vary from minor or temporary skin irritation to very painful inflammation with blisters persisting for several weeks and possibly requiring hospitalization. Two of the most troublesome plants, poison ivy and poison sumac, are shown on pages 86-87.

INTERNAL POISONING

Plants considered as "internal poisons" are those that cause a chemical or physiological disturbance, or death, when eaten. True poisoning of this type, unlike allergies or dermatitis, does not depend on a previous sensitivity of the individual. The term *poisonous* as used here does not necessarily mean "fatal," but that which causes any symptoms of toxicity.

Much folklore surrounds the subject of plant poisoning, yet only a small percentage of all the plants known causes toxic reactions. A few are mildly toxic and a very few can be extremely so and even fatal if eaten in sufficient quantity. Some plants are harmful only if eaten in certain stages of their growth, or only certain parts of the plant may be toxic. Other plants may be poisonous in all stages of development, and all parts may be equally poisonous. Thus the particular type of plant, the stage of growth, the part eaten, the season of the year, the amount eaten, or the condition, age, and size of the person who eats it may all be important factors in determining the potential hazard. To judge from past experiences, "berries," mushrooms, seeds, leaves, stems, flowers, and roots can all be real hazards—particularly to children. Mushrooms are especially treacherous, for some are edible while others are poisonous. The Amanita are deadly. Extreme abdominal pain, profuse vomiting, distorted vision and severe damage to human organs occur if they are eaten.

The table on pages 90-91 gives information on a selected list of plants and their poisonous effects. Following the table some common poisonous plants are illustrated for identification purposes.

In all instances, consult your Poison Control Center, listed often in the telephone directory under "Poison."

Consumer and Community Roles in Poison Control

Poison prevention packaging now is required by law, specifically for dangerous and potentially hazardous household agents as well as many medicines and drugs. These products may be required to be packaged in containers that most children under five years of age will not be able to open, but don't be surprised to learn that there are some children who can circumvent any safety measure and package.

As consumers, we have the power to accept or reject products in order to encourage changes in packaging and in content. Do not buy poisonous products which are packaged in containers likely to attract a child's interest or confuse him about its contents. Complain to store managers about such items and write to the Consumer Product Safety Commission, Washington, D.C. Speak out for products that are safe to use around children.

Too often we buy something not really necessary for household maintenance or yard care. Consider substitutes which may eliminate one source of danger to your child. Ask for information from local garden clubs about how to control undesirable situations in your yard with a minimum use of pesticides, sprays, and chemicals. A constantly filled bird feeder, a thriving community of ladybugs, may offer a safer, more effective, and attractive solution to control of the outdoor insect population than several gallons of sprayed chemicals.

NAME	POISONOUS PARTS	SIGNS AND SYMPTOMS
Arum family: calla lily, dumbcane, elephant's ear	All parts	Severe burning of mucous membranes with swelling of tongue and throat, nausea, vomiting, diarrhea, salivation, rare direct systemic effects
Black locust	Bark, foliage, and seed	Nausea, vomiting, weakness, depression
Bleeding heart or Dutchman's breeches	All parts	Trembling, staggering, respiratory distress, convulsions
Castor bean	Seed (poison, if chewed). If swallowed whole, the hard seed coat prevents absorption and poisoning)	Severe diarrhea and vomiting, convulsions.
Crowfoot family: buttercup, cowslip or marsh marigold, larkspur, monkshood	All parts; for monkshood, especially roots and seeds	Burning sensation of mouth and skin, nausea, vomiting, low blood pressure, weak pulse, convulsions
Deadly nightshade	Berries, leaves, and roots	Fever, rapid heartbeat, dilation of pupils, skin hot, flushed, dry
Elderberry, black and scarlet elder	Leaves, shoots, and bark	Nausea, vomiting, diarrhea
Foxglove	Leaves	Nausea, diarrhea, stomach pain, severe headache, irregular heartbeat and pulse, tremors, convulsions
Poison hemlock	All parts	Diarrhea, nausea, muscular weakness, respiratory paralysis, convulsions
Hyacinth	Bulb	Severe diarrhea, vomiting
Jessamine or yellow jessamine	All parts	Profuse sweating, muscular weakness, convulsions, respiratory depression
Thornapple, jimsonweed, stinkweed	All parts, especially seeds	Thirst, dilation of pupils, dry mouth, red skin, headache, hallucinations, rapid pulse, high blood pressure, delirium, convulsions, coma
Laurel: mountain, black, sheep, American	All parts	Salivation, running eyes and nose, vomiting, convulsions, slowing of pulse, low blood pressure, paralysis

NAME	POISONOUS PARTS	SIGNS AND SYMPTOMS
Lily-of-the-valley	Leaves and flowers	Irregular heartbeat, stomach upset
Mistletoe	Berries	Diarrhea and irregular heartbeat and pulse similar to digitalis
Narcissus family: daffodil, jonquil	Bulb	Diarrhea and vomiting
Nutmeg	Seeds	Hallucinations and elation, stomach pain, red skin, dry mouth, drowsiness, stupor, double vision, delirium. (Two nutmegs can be fatal.)
Oleander	Leaves	Nausea, severe vomiting, stomach pain, dizziness, slowed pulse, irregular heartbeat, marked dilation of pupils, bloody diarrhea, drowsiness, unconsciousness, paralysis of lungs. (One leaf can kill an adult.)
Pokeweed, pokeberry, scoke, inkberry	All parts, especially root	Burning bitter taste in mouth, persistent vomiting, slowed respiration, difficult breathing, weakness, tremors and convulsions. (May be fatal.)
Rhododendron	All parts	Salivation, vomiting, convulsions, slowing of pulse, low blood pressure, paralysis
Rhubarb	Leaves only	Nausea, vomiting, abdominal pain, inability to urinate, hemorrhages
Sweet pea	All parts, but especially seeds	Paralysis, slow and weak pulse, respiratory depression, convulsions
Wisteria	Pods	Severe diarrhea, collapse
Yew	All parts	Diarrhea, dilation of pupils, muscular weakness, coma, convulsions, cardiac and respiratory depression
Mushrooms (*Amanita muscaria and phalloides*)	All parts	Stomach cramps, vomiting, diarrhea, difficult breathing mental disturbance, convulsions and coma

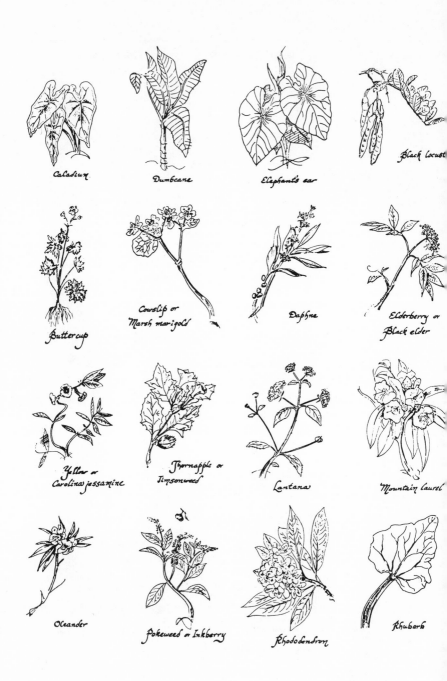

Caladium

Dumbcane

Elephant's ear

Black locust

Buttercup

Cowslip or
Marsh marigold

Daphne

Elderberry or
Black elder

Yellow or
Carolina jessamine

Thornapple or
Jimsonweed

Lantana

Mountain laurel

Oleander

Pokeweed or Inkberry

Rhododendron

Rhubarb

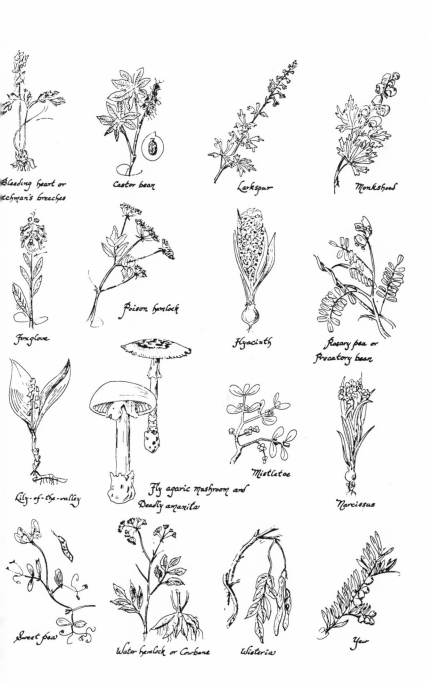

Bleeding heart or Dutchman's breeches

Castor bean

Larkspur

Monkshood

Foxglove

Poison hemlock

Hyacinth

Rosary pea or Precatory bean

Lily-of-the-valley

Fly agaric mushroom and Deadly amanita

Mistletoe

Narcissus

Sweet pea

Water hemlock or Cowbane

Wisteria

Yew

Community efforts to reduce the number of childhood poisonings often take the form of organizing and supporting a poison control center. Such centers have access to information about almost any toxic or potentially toxic product and the specific antidotes required for proper treatment. A phone call to a poison control center can make available immediate first-aid instructions. Some centers are equipped only to supply information; most give treatment as well. Usually sponsored by professional groups such as community or state health departments, medical schools, or medical societies, poison control centers can provide many communities with the impetus to engage in educational and *prevention* activities at the local level which, in the long run, represent the most effective solution to the problem of childhood poisonings.

Other primary sources of immediate help are personal physicians, pharmacists, nurses, and hospital emergency rooms.

MOTOR-POWERED VEHICLES

7

Automobiles*

Automotive collisions are the most common cause of accidental injuries during childhood. Each year more than 2700 children, from infancy to the age of 15, are killed while they are riding in automobiles. Injuries number in the tens of thousands, many of which result in permanent disabilities. A great many of these deaths and injuries can be prevented or reduced.

Small children require special restraining devices in automobiles because of their undeveloped physical structure. Lap belts alone can possibly cause internal injuries when a crash occurs, although safety experts agree that safety belts are the single most effective device currently available for adults and older children. Some diagonal shoulder belts also are not suitable for small children. This should be specified in your car manual. If, however, no special child safety device is available, a standard belt, positioned low across the hips, below the child's stomach, should be used. This is far safer than letting the child ride loose or in mother's lap.

Children's car seats are not simply positioning devices intended to keep the child confined and able to see out of windows. The purpose of using car seats is to provide crash protection, if an accident occurs.

* Portions of the text and the illustration of car seats are used with the permission of *Physicians for Automotive Safety*, Irvington, N.J.

In spite of government safety requirements in effect since 1971, many children's car seats and harnesses give inadequate protection. Effective crash protection is available through the use of devices that have been subjected to actual tests. The government standard has not specified such testing.

The following specific types of devices are suggested:

1. *For the infant:* Infant Carriers are designed to face rearward or sideways. The baby rides in a semi-upright position, secured with a harness. The carrier is held down with a lap belt.

2. *For the child able to sit up without support*: The Shield is preferred especially for children up to the age of two or three. In the event of a crash the child's body is caught by the padding shield which acts as a cushion. The shield is anchored with a lap belt and no harness is needed. But if your child is overly active and hard to discipline, he or she may climb out or slide through while you are driving. Consider this before you make a choice.

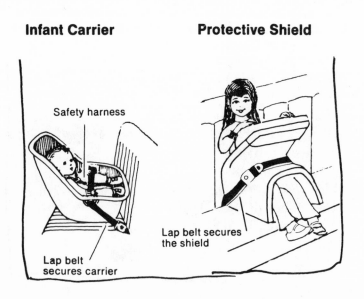

Infant Carrier   **Protective Shield**

Safety harness

Lap belt
secures carrier

Lap belt secures
the shield

The Traditional Style Car Seat: The child is held by a harness which consists of two shoulder straps, a lap belt, and crotch straps. The seat itself is strapped down with a vehicle lap belt. Some devices require the belt to be threaded through the back where it can remain permanently buckled. Others must be fastened with the belt around the front of the seat after the child has been buckled into the harness. If the seat has no raised side panels to keep the belt from pressing into the child's body, the belt must be threaded through the back. A number of seats require additional anchorage: A strap leading from the top must be hooked into the tongue portion of the lap belt in the seat behind (this makes one set of belts unusable) or, if the device is used in the back of a sedan, the strap hooks into an anchorage assembly bolted to the rear window ledge.

The Safety Harness: Effective protection is provided at low cost, but permanent installation is necessary. The child may sit on a firm cushion.

Traditional Car Seat   Safety Harness

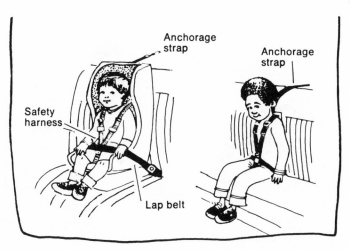

Whichever device is selected, **correct installation and use are vital**. Manufacturer's instructions on installing the devices and securing the child in it must be conscientiously followed.

1. A seat designed to be used with a top anchorage strap must be used in this way every time. Even if it seems that the seat is held securely enough with just the vehicle lap belt, this is not so. The violent forces unleashed in a crash would tip the seat forward or even cause it to break, slamming your child's head into the instrument panel.

2. The device must be strapped down as tightly as possible with the vehicle lap belt. If it is used in the front seat of a car with joined lap and shoulder belts, instructions on where to place the shoulder strap must also be carefully followed.

3. If a harness is provided, this must be used each time because even in a minor mishap the child would otherwise be thrown out of the safety seat. A number of forward-facing seats for the older child adjust to a reclining position for the child's comfort. For maximum safety, however, a fully upright position is recommended.

Children over the age of four, weighing at least 40 pounds, should be placed on a firm cushion, two or three inches high, and strapped in with the lap belt while sitting upright against the back of the car seat. The belt must be pulled snug to prevent it riding up across the abdomen. Do not strap two children into one belt. This makes a proper fit impossible.

A shoulder belt also should be used so long as it crosses the child's chest, but not the neck or face. (See your Car Owner's Manual for recommendations.) A shoulder belt must not be used without a lap belt by anyone—child or adult.

Parents are often concerned that their children will dislike riding restrained. A child who has been used to riding with restraints from an early age will continue to accept them as a matter of course with only occasional protests. A child who has been allowed to romp around the car may object at first to being strapped in. A lot will depend on your determination. Don't start the car until everyone is buckled up, including yourself and all other passengers.

Children quickly learn to sleep sitting upright in their safety seats. They can be made more comfortable with the help of a pillow.

It is not harmful for infants to ride in a half upright position. For a newborn, pad the container well and wedge a rolled-up blanket around the baby's head and shoulders to keep the head supported.

On long trips make frequent stops and give your child a chance to exercise. A baby should be taken out of the carrier and laid flat to allow stretching and kicking. Be sure to pull into a rest area or well off the highway.

When choosing a device, parents will want to buy the safest available, but careful thought should be given to installation requirements. Also taken into consideration should be: (1) age and temperament of the child; (2) number of children needing special restraints; (3) number of other family members; and (4) size and type of vehicle owned (sedan, station wagon, camper).

Cargo and toys may be dangerous. Lawnmowers, bicycles, luggage, or sharp objects carried unsecured inside the vehicle present a hazard. The only safe place for cargo is in the trunk or on a roof rack. Do not allow your children to play with pens, pencils, or metal toys while the car is moving. There is no way the cargo area of a station wagon can be made safe for children.

Remember also that unrestrained passengers not only risk their own lives but could injure others who are belted in. So always insist that everyone is buckled up.

You should refer to *current* reviews in consumer magazines for evaluation of devices on the market. In addition excellent current information about automotive safety is available from the Physicians for Automotive Safety, Irvington, New Jersey. This private organization is active in evaluating comparative merits of these devices. It will provide prompt responses to requests for product advice.

Having accomplished suitable restraining approaches, you also need to consider your children's behavior in automobiles. Distractions because of arguments, jumping around, throwing things, putting head or arms out of the windows, all increase accident potential. Provide suitable toys or other distractions for your children which will keep their movements to a minimum. On long trips, include frequent stops to stretch and go to the bathroom. *Finally, remember: mother's lap is not safe, nor a substitute for a safety device.*

Your own driving behavior is also crucial to your children's safety. This topic is discussed on pp. 154-155, "When Adults Put Their Children in Danger."

Other Motor Vehicles

Minibikes are recreational vehicles designed for riding on backwoods trails or open fields. They vary in power from that of a lawnmower to that of a highly tuned trail bike, the usual power range being from 5 to 10 horsepower. They are able to attain speeds of 30 to 50 miles per hour on the open trail. Clearly such a device is not a toy. If a parent cannot convey this distinction to his child, the use of a minibike should not be allowed.

Minibikes in most states cannot be legally driven on public roads and do not require registration or licenses. This fact plus their small size makes minibikes very popular among eight- to sixteen-year-old children.

Once you agree to your child's use of a minibike, you

have the responsibility to make sure that your child knows how to handle the bike. Do not buy the machine and simply turn your child loose with it. He must be trained to use the controls properly, to manipulate them automatically: stop and go, gear changes, riding in circles; figure 8's and panic stops.

A safety helmet should always be worn. A condition you can lay down for use of the minibike is: *Wear that helmet or else.* Other protective clothing includes boots or sturdy shoes, heavy long pants, a long-sleeved shirt, and gloves. Goggles or a face shield are also a good idea.

Since minibikes are restricted in most states to off-the-road locations, your child soon tires of going around in circles in the backyard. The best and safest places are dirt or grass trails specifically designated for minibikes and under adult supervision. Any off-the-road area not designated for minibikes should be inspected for hazards.

The most serious hazard to the minibiker—and one that can be lethal—is an inadvertent collision with a wire

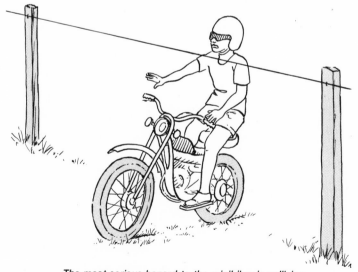

The most serious hazard to the minibiker is collision with a wire or cable, at dusk or at night.

or cable in his path, producing severe neck injuries. This type of accident occurs particularly at dusk when visibility is poor. It is imperative that medical care be obtained immediately.

Other hazards include potholes, fallen branches, creek beds, and show-off behavior.

If your child has a minibike, you should know how to operate it, also. Both of you should know how to maintain and service the vehicle regularly.

Motorcycles, scooters, dune buggies, and **snowmobiles** present safety hazards similar to those associated with autos and minibikes. Proper regulations as well as protective helmets and clothing are needed.

Some accidents are due to mechanical failure, such as brakes failing or a throttle that sticks open. Others, however, are due to human error. Stunting, excessive speed, and collision with fixed or moving objects are associated with many of these accidents. As with minibikes, the use of designated and supervised trails offers the best protection.

SWIMMING: SAFETY HABITS

8

Drowning is the second most common cause of death for children between five and fourteen years of age. Most drownings in this age group involve inadequate or careless adult supervision.

Children should be taught to float as early as possible (see bathtub water exercises for babies as described on pp. 49-50). Swimming instructions should wait until at least three years of age. Under three, the child's head is large in proportion to the rest of his body, making it more difficult for him to hold his head out of the water to breathe. In addition, you cannot count on the very young child to retain swimming skills unless there is frequent practice. Although you may want to give swimming instructions to your child under three years of age, remember that a child of this maturity should never be considered water-safe, no matter how skillful he seems to be.

Exposure to an environment which allows water play will prepare your child for learning to swim. Early play in a bathtub or wading pools and practice in breathing skills will help him enjoy himself and gradually feel secure.

Once your child is comfortable in the water and is at an appropriate age, group swimming lessons can often be beneficial. The fun of being with other children and the opportunity to observe the skill or lack of it in other beginners often will motivate him to keep trying. Classes which have from 6 to 12 children allow instructors sufficient time with each child. More and more communities have such classes available at low cost through the Red Cross, neighborhood pool clubs, Y-groups (YM-WCA; YM-WHA), and other organizations oriented to recreation safety.

You should encourage your child's learning to swim by praise and play. The youngster who is encouraged to have fun with Mom and Dad in the water will go to the next lesson with a greater sense of his own ability and security. Skill and competence will take time to develop.

Home and community swimming pools are associated with three major causes of accidents. These are: falling on slippery surfaces such as walks, decks, diving boards, ladders; colliding with the bottom or sides of the pool because of insufficient depth for sliding or diving; drowning when swimming alone.

Teaching your child proper poolside behavior is extremely important. Pushing, running, stunting, and gen-

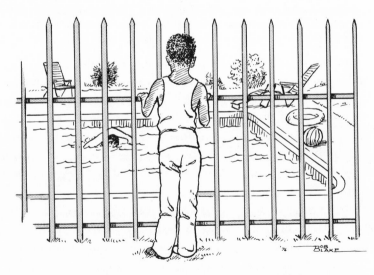

Swimming pools should be fenced on all sides.

erally showing off must be prohibited. Energy should be channeled to safe water games and friendly competition under appropriate supervision.

Swimming pools should be fenced on all sides with barriers that are difficult to climb. Shock hazards should be eliminated by keeping all electrically-operated equipment in good repair. TV, radios, loudspeaker systems, and other equipment brought to the pool should remain at a safe distance away from the water and pool area.

Ponds, lakes, and sounds attract children and you must see to it that their dangers are avoided. Make sure that these water areas are free of whirlpools and fast currents. The water in which your child will swim should be clear enough for you visually to check the depth (unless you know beforehand), as well as any dangerous objects on the bottom.

Ocean swimming can be especially hazardous. Children can learn how to swim in pools, but learning how to apply swimming skills to the ocean is a new experience. Ocean swimmers must remember that the water is in constant motion, even on very calm days. This constant motion can cause a variety of potential hazards such as undertow, cross-currents, rip-tides, and run-outs. Guarded beaches with competent lifeguards are the safest places for ocean swimming. But even there, you must be alert. Toddlers are very easily knocked down by surf and pulled by undertow. Follow the advice of lifeguards about water conditions. Maintain supervision of your own children even when a lifeguard is present. Even strong swimmers should stay within effective rescue range, approximately 100 yards from the shore.

You should teach your children what to do if they do get into trouble in the water. When pulled away from the shore, teach them to relax and try to swim at an angle toward the shore, across the current, until free of the pulling effect. Your child may drift parallel to the shore

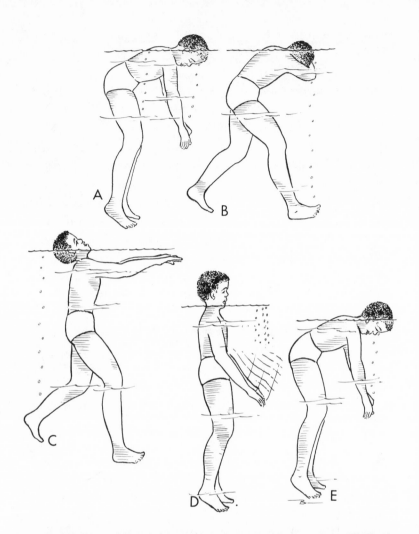

(A) With lungs full, float face down with back of neck on surface. (B) Slowly lift arms and cross them in front of forehead, as if to ward off a blow. Get ready for downward thrust. (C) Exhale through nose while raising head until mouth is in the air, shoulders underwater. (D) With head vertical, thrust downward gently with arms while inhaling through mouth. (E) With lungs full, drop head forward and return to position (A), arms to sides. Relax. If necessary, use gentle scissors kick to return to surface. Learners rest three seconds here; experts, ten seconds.

As you perfect the bobbing technique, practice tilting your body, aiming towards shore and giving frog or scissors kicks, continuing the bobbing actions until you reach safety. If you get tired, go back to the vertical position until you feel rested. Bobbing is drownproof!

but should be able to make his way to land even if it is at a distance from where he entered the water.

Another technique all parents and children should learn is often referred to as drownproofing. This is essentially floating almost motionless with air-filled lungs, face in the water, then bobbing up with face out to exhale and inhale. This procedure is repeated rhythmically as shown in the illustration. The caption provides description of the procedures.

FIRES IN THE HOME

9

Every year a startling number of babies and young children die or are injured in fires. Careless smoking and children playing with matches and cigarette lighters cause one out of every five fires. Don't tempt children by leaving matches and igniting fuels or devices, such as cigarette lighters, around the house.

Never leave children alone in a house, without adult supervision. In minutes they can kindle a fire to trap them. Children panic in fires and, when you or other responsible adults are not there to supervise them, they have been known to do foolish things like hide under beds or in closets.

Home fire drills are excellent safety measures. The best way for your child not to panic in case of fire is for him to know what he is going to do *before* a fire ever breaks out.

Your child's first impulse in a fire should always be *escape*. Too many people become unnecessary fire victims because they sadly underestimate the killing power and speed of fire and smoke.

Every family member should know how to escape quickly, preferably by two routes in case one is blocked. Practice your escape plan with all members of the family. Make sure everyone knows what to do and where to go. Have a central meeting place identified—such as a neighbor's house or the nearest street corner or alarm box. As you evacuate your family to a specific location, tell some one—neighbors—to call the fire department (do

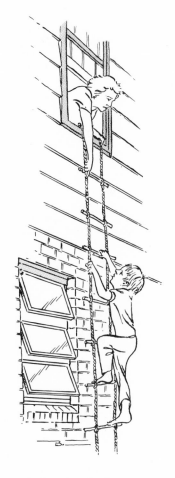

Every family member should know how to escape quickly from fire in the home, preferably by two routes in the event that one is blocked.

not stay in the house to call), or have him use the nearest alarm box.

Full skirts on little girls and flowing sleeves on house-coats are highly flammable. Wool and fiberglass are the safest fabrics for clothes. Untreated cotton and some of the synthetics are the most dangerous. *If a child's clothing should catch on fire*, teach him the *drop and roll technique*. Have him cross his arms across his chest so that his right hand touches his left shoulder and his left hand touches his right shoulder. Then have him drop to the floor or on the ground. Tell him to roll over and over slowly. Wrap a rug around him if available. Lying down and folding his arms will keep the flames away from his face; rolling over will help cut off the air and put out the fire. Impress upon your child: *never run!* That lets more air get to the flames, which then burn faster than ever.

Families should have some reliable fire-fighting equipment. Fire extinguishers or several garden hoses with strategically located outlets are valuable. If the fire is very small and has just started, you can possibly extinguish it yourself with the proper equipment at hand. In any case, always send the children outside the house. Smoke, not flames, is the real killer in a fire. According to some studies, as many as 80 percent of fire-related deaths are due to inhaling poisonous fumes long before the flames ever reach the victim.

Smoke detectors, along with heat detectors, are among your best fire safety investments. A smoke detector located between a family asleep and the rest of the home is the minimum recommendation of fire protection authorities. Heat or smoke detectors are also advised in all other major areas of your home, particularly in your living room, where most fires begin because of careless cigarette smoking.

With three-quarters of fires occurring at night, a warning alarm could save your lives by giving you some head start. The smoke detector could give you this alarm before a slow-burning fire in bedding or upholstery generated sufficient heat to activate a heat detector. You could be unconscious before the heat alarm went off. Your household warning equipment must respond to both extremes: rapidly developing high heat fire plus the smoke and deadly gasses produced by slow, smoldering fire.

Test your detectors against all household equipment which might be in full operation at night. Will they be heard over the sound of an air-conditioner or room-humidifier? All alarm-sounding devices should have a minimum rating of 85 decibels at 10 feet.

Regularly test your equipment to be sure it is functioning properly. Set aside a definite day each week for the test. Make sure your detector has been certified by a recognized testing laboratory and that your unit comes with maintenance instructions as well as replacement and service information. Ask your supplier or installing contractor where to obtain repair or replacement service and where and how parts requiring replacement can be obtained within no more than two weeks. If feasible, arrange a maintenance contract with the installer.

Grease and food fires can be avoided by never leaving unattended on a stove or a table-top oven such things as lard, cooking oil, bacon, and other meat fat. Do not allow grease to collect on stove surfaces and under burners. Keep ovens and burners clean and free of grease build-up. *Grease fires cannot be extinguished with water.* Small fires contained in a pan can be extinguished by cutting off oxygen to the fire. Cover the pan with a pot lid, wet towel, or a thick wet pad of newspapers; if handy, grab a box of baking soda or salt and smother the fire with either. If the burning grease has spread from the pan to other parts of the stove or curtains or walls, a dry chemical extinguisher should be used if available.

An all-purpose type of fire extinguisher for use on fires caused by burning liquids such as grease or oil as well as electrical fires is best. Buy reliable equipment that carries the label of the Underwriters Laboratories (UL) or Factory Mutual (FM). Read the instructions so that you know automatically what to do in operating the fire extinguisher.

Electrical fires are especially dangerous. Such fires may smolder unnoticed until flames flare up. Avoidance of such fires can be accomplished by preventive measures such as:

Buy electrical equipment and cords which carry the UL label.

Replace broken and frayed cords.

Do not overload circuits or extensions (Consult an electrician or your local Building Inspection Department and have him check the wiring and circuits.)

Know where your switchbox is and how to replace proper fuses or reset switches.

Know how to pull the main switch(es) to turn off all electricity in your house, if you do not know how to turn off the particular circuit that is causing the trouble.

Have a *working* flashlight available at all times. Check the batteries periodically.

If an electrical fire occurs, do not use water. Pull the main switch in the switchboard to cut off electrical current. Use a dry chemical fire extinguisher *and call the fire department immediately.*

Flammable liquids, such as gasoline, oil, and solvents don't necessarily start open flames to begin burning. Their fumes are often flammable and can travel for some distance to a near-by open flame. Therefore, they should be stored in a safe area, well-ventilated to avoid fume buildup, away from pilot lights and electrical equipment. Never use them around flames, sparks, or anything hot. Never use gasoline to start fires. The flames can move quickly up to your clothing. Most important, keep the containers covered tightly and locked away where children cannot get to them. Also, rags or paper saturated with these liquids should always be discarded and never be kept after use.

If you must transport gasoline or any other quickly flammable liquid in containers in your car, be sure that children do not accompany you and that no container leakage can occur during the transport.

Do not overlook potential danger in storage sheds, garages, utility rooms where mowers, motorcycles, motorbikes and other equipment using gasoline fuel are stored. Children playing with matches in such places have been badly injured or killed when flammable vapors or leaking gasoline have exploded.

All heat fires should be contained in their proper places, and open fires, such as in fireplaces, should have safety screens. Combustibles such as paper, cloth, leaves, rubbish, oily rags, wood shavings, should be kept away from heat and from such ignition sources as heaters, fireplaces, furnaces, ranges, and electrical equipment, including even lighted bulbs. Dispose of all trash promptly.

Special care should be taken in handling heat-producing electrical appliances, since they continue to hold heat for some time after they have been turned off. Remember not to leave hot irons and dangling cords from irons, percolators, skillets, lamps, where children can reach them. Electric fans, heaters, and vaporizers should also be kept out of a child's reach. Provide a safety screen in front of such appliances or cover them with a fireproof mesh, so little fingers can't get in.

FIREARMS: DANGERS TO CHILDREN

10

When firearms, such as guns, are present in a home, children are in danger. Most firearm accidents involving children occur when:

1. Guns are improperly stored.
2. Children play with the guns which they have found.
3. Adult supervision is lacking.

Accidents frequently occur when guns are being cleaned by adults in the presence of other people, or when they are being shown to other people. These accidents happen as often indoors as outdoors. Many children injured or killed are innocent bystanders, but sometimes the gun has been playfully aimed at them. Another child is most often the person who pulls the trigger.

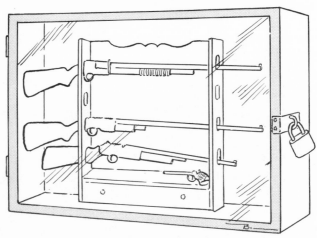

Guns should be kept in a locked cabinet to which children will have no possible access.

The only effective protection for children against gun accidents is following absolutely all safety precautions. Guns should be kept in a locked cabinet to which children will have *no possible access*. (Be sure the keys are also inaccessible.) All guns should be unloaded before being locked away. Ammunition should be stored separately from guns, also in locked cabinets. Safety devices are available which prevent firing until the device is removed. Guns should be cleaned in an area away from other people, particularly children.

If you expect to use a gun, carry it unloaded to the place where it will be fired. Use guns in areas designated for such purposes and observe all safety rules. Gun accidents in such areas usually involve shooting at something that has been mistaken for the correct target; safety catch not in use; carrying a loaded gun while climbing over obstacles like a stone wall or barbed wire fence; lifting a loaded weapon from trucks, cars, and boats.

If you are a hunter, protect your children in your own home and on trips by observing gun safety rules at all times. Teach them to avoid situations where guns are available without your presence. Impress on your child never to play with another child who has a gun in his possession. Tell him that he must immediately leave if he encounters someone with a gun and report to you promptly the circumstances. (Even though the gun may be a toy, it is better to be fooled than sorry.)

SAFETY IN THE NATURAL ENVIRONMENT 11

Yard Safety

Power Mowers and Tractors

Lawn mowers are designed to cut and will do just that to anything in their path including the human body. Four major accident patterns are associated with power lawn mowers. These are:

1. Contact with a moving blade.
2. Propelled object striking a bystander.
3. Mowers overturning when in use, particularly on steep slopes.
4. Mower running over a person.

Ignorance and carelessness are the chief factors in these accidents. Young children should never be permitted to operate power lawn mowers, whether the hand-type or riding-type. Older children should receive careful instructions in the proper use of the machine. Continued supervision by adults is essential until the older child demonstrates skill and awareness of the need for constant vigilance.

When purchasing a power mower, look for the following safety features:

1. Rear guard to prevent feet or hands from coming in contact with rotating blades.
2. Discharge opening aimed downward or provided

with a deflector plate to attach when grass-catcher is not in use.

3. Engine exhaust located on side opposite discharge opening to prevent backfire sparks from igniting grass-catching bag.

4. Handle up-stops to prevent handles from rising when mower hits an obstacle.

5. Written safety instruction booklet and precaution labels on the machine.

Once you have proper familiarity with the machine, it is essential to prepare the area to be mowed. All debris, both natural and man-made, should be raked off. Most power lawn mowers have rotary blades. These blades can reach speeds of 200 miles an hour and can hurl objects such as rocks and twigs 50 feet and further. When even small objects are propelled with such great force, severe injury can result if they strike a person. *Children and other people (and pets) should be kept away from the area that is being mowed.*

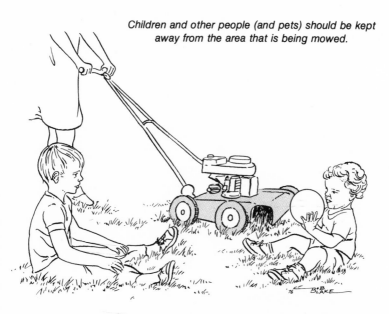

Children and other people (and pets) should be kept away from the area that is being mowed.

Whoever is mowing should wear sturdy shoes—never barefoot or with sandals. Always turn off the mower when:

- you leave it
- you unclog or adjust it
- you refuel it

Never refuel a mower:

- indoors
- when the motor is running
- while you are smoking

Farm tractors are the major cause of fatal and permanently crippling accidents in agricultural areas. Parents on farms have a special responsibility to instruct their children in their proper use. Parents themselves must also strictly observe recommended safety precautions when operating all farm machinery.

More than half of all tractor accidents are the result of the tractor overturning. This is most often caused by loss of control due to high speed operation, climbing steep banks, and collision with hidden obstructions such as tree stumps, ditches, and large rocks. Brakes also are often misused.

In addition to observing safety rules, tractor owners can obtain extra protection by attaching a protective frame or crush-resistant cab and seat belts. These hold and encircle the operator and will prevent crushing injuries in the event of an overturn.

Camping, Hiking, and Back Packing

Camping, hiking, and backpacking are activities which are attracting more and more families. People are seeking the solitude and beauty of natural areas. Parents want their children to have the fun of being in the woods. Children imagine scenes of Daniel Boone, pioneers, and discoverers of new lands. The pleasures of such adventures need to be encouraged. While the patterns of safety suggested for use in other settings are applicable, some specific additional preparations should be made for camping, hiking, and backpacking.

Outings in well-traveled country for short periods of time may be dealt with more simply than extended trips into remote areas. If you are sure you will never be far from help, routine precautions which are really intended to enhance general comfort may be sufficient. Clothing appropriate for the weather, nourishment, insect repellant may be all that is needed.

However, experienced outdoorsmen and professionals such as park rangers know that people, and particularly children, often wander farther away from civilization than they planned. This fact suggests that even on the shortest hike, some device should be carried so that you can signal for help. A metal pocket mirror can be used to flash signals when the sun is shining. Waterproof matches can be used to start a smoky signal fire. A shrill whistle is easy to use and carry. For even short trips in well-traveled areas let someone know where you are going and when to expect your return. Small children should be accompanied by adults or *remain within sight of adults*. Children become absorbed in play and may wander great distances. In wooded areas confusion and panic happen quickly. Teach your children to "stay together."

If you and your children have not had experience with living in remote areas under primitive conditions, do so only after properly informing yourselves of the safest techniques. Books are available on the subject. Clubs in many communities can provide helpful advice and may even organize inexpensive trips led by experienced guides. If you do go into remote areas:

- Let someone who is remaining behind know your itinerary and when you expect to return.
- Pace yourself in accordance with your physical condition and with the temperature and the conditions of the trail.
- Carry adequate food and fluids.
- Carry and know how to use first aid gear.
- Know basic first aid as taught by the American Red Cross and discussed at some length in this book.
- Know what to wear for comfort and safety. Prefer wool clothing. It is best to wear layers of clothing for maximum warmth and comfort.
- Understand that, because of the remote situation, if injury occurs first aid may have to be replaced with specific emergency treatment usually not included in routine first aid courses.
- Remember that "feeling chilled" can be the danger sign of *hypothermia*—a dangerous condition which occurs when the body loses heat faster than it produces it. Get your child out of any wind or breeze; thoroughly dry him; and use dry wool clothing or wrapping on him. Crawl into a sleeping bag with your child. Your body warmth can be effective in restoring heat to his body.

The physical condition of each family member should be reviewed. Plan a trip appropriate for each person's age and level of physical activity prior to the trip. Everyone's stamina will be challenged and strained by unaccustomed circumstances.

A detailed understanding of the weather as well as of the natural environment in which you will travel is vital. A check of up-to-the minute weather conditions at the time of departure can be made through offices of state or local police, local weather stations, forest service personnel, or forest rangers. Hazardous weather conditions occur in many forms. Extreme cold subjects people to exposure and frostbite. Heavy continuous rain, in addition to personal discomfort and possibly dangerous body heat loss, may cause earth and rock slides, obliterate trails, flood ditches and creeks.

Lightning can cause injury and death. Don't get under an isolated tree or near wirefences or other metallic conductors of electricity, such as golf clubs. Your best bet is to take shelter inside a building or in thick woods, or to drop to your knees, bend forward, and put hands on knees if you are caught in an open area. If an enclosed car is available, get into it. Do not touch a tree during a storm; if the bark is wet, it will conduct electricity. Never stay in water, pools or lakes, when lightning occurs, or in ditches or hollows where water may be present.

Determine what special equipment you should carry to assure safety and enjoyment under normal as well as emergency conditions. For example, for a three-day overnight hike on a national trail which provides shelters, sleeping bags would be necessary but a tent would not. However, for an emergency circumstance in which you were unable to reach the shelter, how would you protect yourself? Compact gear is available for such situations.

Typical hazards associated with outdoor living can be avoided. Tents are made of either flammable fabric or flame-resistant fabric. *No tent is flameproof.* All sources of flame must be kept away from the tent fabric. This includes candles, fuel-fired stoves, fueled lanterns, and heaters. Campfires should be built downwind from the tent and several yards away. All campfires should be completely extinguished before leaving camp or when going to sleep. Don't smoke near sleeping bags.

Try to anticipate the situations which could transform pleasure into agony. Preparing for the unexpected can help you if you are faced with unpleasant circumstances.

Teach your children both the delights and dangers of such outings. Help them to understand their role in having a happy time as well as their part in any emergency which may occur. Just as your children should know how to react when there is a fire or accident in the home, so too must they know how to behave in the natural environment.

Camps

Camps can be safe and healthful environments for your children if there is adequate supervision by a sufficient number of experienced personnel. Whether a camp is near water, mountains, or other kind of setting seems to have little to do with accident experience. Most important are human behavior factors. The camp personnel and the campers should recognize the following as times at which accidents are more likely to occur:

- When participation in an activity demands a great deal beyond the camper's normal energy or physical strength and endurance (for example, long hikes or swims).
- When there is insufficient adult supervision (for example, unqualified personnel).
- Just before mid-day and evening meals (when hungry and tired).

Most accidents which occur at camp are usually minor, but some can be serious. Prevention of those accidents that occur often involves sticking to the camp rules in general and to basic preventive measures.

An important part of any camp safety program is quick and effective first aid facilities, with qualified medical personnel on site or within quick call for prompt treatment and care.

Safe and sanitary facilities, such as cabins, kitchens, etc., are important.

Kite Flying

Every spring, thousands of youngsters take to the outdoors to enjoy one of the great seasonal sports—kite flying. And, every spring, a few of them end up with bruises, broken bones, or even worse.

Kite flying is fun. But unless a few simple rules are observed, it can also be dangerous. Here are some things you should know (and some things you can tell your children) to help make kite flying safer:

- Make sure the area where kites are flown is far from electric power lines, TV and radio antennas.
- Do not use wire or metal in building a kite. Use only wood, paper and cloth.
- Make sure the kite string does not have a metallic thread. This type of string could result in a serious electrical shock if it comes into contact with an electric power line.
- If the kite becomes entangled in a power line, leave it there. Do not try to pull it free or attempt to climb the pole.
- Make sure the kite string is dry, and avoid flying kites when there is lightning.

Power lines have become so commonplace that parents and children sometimes forget that the electricity they carry can be dangerous. Also, serious disruptions of electric power to a community can occur because of certain types of kites getting entangled in power lines.

SAFETY IN THE COMMUNITY

12

Pedestrian and Traffic Safety

Children are not capable of behaving in traffic the way an adult should. Children under the age of ten, and perhaps a few years older, *cannot comprehend a traffic situation as a whole*, made up as it is of a complex combination of events and activities: seeing, hearing, judging distance, estimating time needed to go from one corner to another, guessing what the vehicle drivers will do.

Children must be taught to behave safely as pedestrians and bicyclists. The degree of responsibility they may be expected to assume for their own safety must be built up gradually. From the toddler who requires absolute protection in traffic, the child must change to a person able to protect himself. To do this, as the child gradually matures physically and emotionally, you must provide him with appropriate information and example, and the child must gain experience in using this acquired knowledge.

Many parents and other adults, such as teachers, do not fully realize what can be expected of children in traffic situations and therefore how much information children can absorb about traffic safety. Tots, five and under, should not be out of sight of adults wherever there are parked cars or moving traffic. When crossing streets small children should be held firmly by the hand. When crossing with a baby carriage or stroller, step out first and

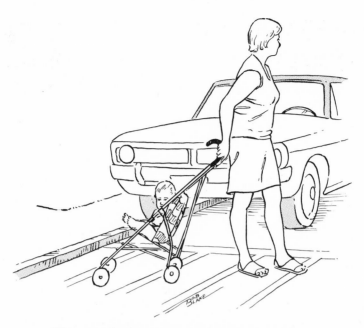

When crossing with a baby carriage or stroller, step out first and pull the carriage after you so you can check the traffic situation.

pull the carriage after you so that you can check the traffic situation.

Do not allow small children to play outdoors without adult supervision wherever there are parked cars and moving traffic. Even though you have forbidden a child to do certain things, *expect him to forget*. Children forget easily, become involved in their play world, and do not necessarily deliberately disobey. They do not have the capacity to make use of complex traffic information automatically until they are at least ten years old. Never call a child from another side of the street or road: walk over and bring him across. When you transport children somewhere in a vehicle, make sure they get in or out only after the vehicle is parked and only on the side away from traffic.

Schools

School itself is a relatively safe place to be. Accident rates during school hours are lower than for other times of the day. The most common injuries in school settings are cuts, lacerations, sprains, and fractures. Most of these are due to carelessness while playing, running, fighting, tripping, in the building or on the playground.

When injuries do occur within a school's jurisdiction, these tend to be much less severe than nonschool-related injuries. There are two major reasons for this favorable experience: the physical building and premises generally exclude many hazards; schooling is a highly supervised experience.

You have responsibility to assist the school officials and teachers in maintaining this favorable experience. School attendance usually begins around the age of five or six. A major contribution to safety at school can be made if you prepare your children to be cooperative. In discussions with professional educators about safety, the child's cooperation and obedience to rules were mentioned as most important ingredients for the implementation of specific safety measures. Fire drills, tornado drills, bus regulations, all are designed to assure safety. Less dramatic but equally important safety programs include playground behavior, proper use of equipment, and behavior during special events such as field trips.

Vocational and industrial art shops can be hazardous areas in schools. Most students begin such programs by learning about the hazards and how to avoid them. Improper use of equipment, disregard of prescribed procedures, and lack of consideration of fellow classmates are involved in a large number of these accidents. Such programs are generally available to students not younger than eleven. By that time, your child should have developed a high degree of self-control, a sense of mutual respect for his fellow students, and a willingness to obey rules and regulations. Without these characteristics your child can do himself and other people great physical and social harm, and miss important learning opportunities.

While the primary function of school is education, this must be carried out in a safe, healthful environment. A clearly defined program for dealing with illness and accidents must be part of such an environment. You should become informed about both specific and general school safety programs, assist in the development of needed programs, and volunteer to serve in such programs when necessary. This personal involvement is good for the child and for you in developing an early, solid, and meaningful relationship towards safety goals.

Children going to school must begin to take some responsibility for their own traffic safety. Parents and teachers, however, must continue to recognize the limits of the child's capacities. Children must be made aware of and concerned about traffic situations. Some school systems conduct work shops for teachers, suggesting learning opportunities which can help children understand why we must have traffic safety rules. Children need to develop attitudes at an early age through which they accept and make use of these rules. Two of the most widely used school traffic safety instruction programs are *School Safety Patrols* and the *Safest Route Home Project* made available by the *American Automobile Association* (AAA).

School safety patrol programs use older and reliable students to help other children avoid traffic hazards. The basic responsibility of safety patrols is to remind others about safety rules learned at school as well as at home. For many children, seeing a safety patrol at a designated location warns and reminds them of potential dangers and appropriate behavior. Other children will need specific reminders to wait for the light, to cross at supervised intersections, or to follow any other rules necessary for pedestrian safety. School personnel, often in cooperation with local police and civic groups, instruct and supervise safety patrols. The school children are taught to cooperate with patrols at all times. Patrol members usually wear white belts and badges which identify patrols to other children as well as motorists. Cooperation and compliance with directions given by safety patrols are essential if these patrols are to assure the safety of your children.

If your school does not have a safety patrol, find out why. Your constructive inquiry and help can enhance school officials' efforts to develop similar programs.

A newer program than safety patrols is the Safest Route to School project. This program is designed and offered by the AAA to help schools teach children safe walking habits. In addition, potential hazards along what may appear to be a safe route are reviewed. Parents are asked to participate by approving a specific route. Identification of the safest route is done through discussion and through mapping. *The combination of talking about as well as visualizing* the route has proven to be effective in gaining the active cooperation of the children to *use* the safest route. While specific traffic conditions vary from community to community, several principles underly the Safest Route Home program and are universally applicable. These include:

- Use of most direct safe route.
- Minimum use of road ways, complicated intersections, and intersections with large numbers of turning or crossing vehicles.
- Maximum use of protected intersections including those with police, crossing-guard or safety patrol supervision as well as mechanical traffic controls.
- Selection of routes which converge and bring as

many children together as possible for supervised crossing.

Once a route to and from school is identified, certain hazards will remain. Waiting for buses should be done in a safe area, back from the road. Young children need supervision during this time. Older children often are not interested in supervising younger ones, and an adult may be needed.

For rural and suburban areas, children need special instructions and frequent reminders about walking facing the traffic. While children should respect property along their route, they should understand that their protection comes first and that they should make use of private property to step away from traffic, particularly when there is snow or ice on the road.

Children in urban areas should use sidewalks. They should understand and use safety controls such as traffic lights and crosswalks. Parents can do many things to enhance sidewalk safety. Two effective parent programs that are in use in several areas include block parent programs and parent patrols.

These programs have been started to protect children from child molesters, harassment by older children, fights, and traffic. Block parent programs include specific homes and parents along the entire route from home to school. Some locally agreed upon symbol which is known to the children, law enforcement personnel, and school officials is displayed. Block parents expect to be at home during those times of the day when children will be passing by. The children know that any such parent offers a refuge from any kind of encounter or problem with which the child may want help. Block parent programs often act as a deterrent, thus preventing many incidents. When called upon for help, block parents most often simply get in touch with the school or parents who then take charge of the frightened child.

Parent patrols are active in some heavily populated urban areas. Where large apartment buildings dominate streets, block parents may not be suitable. These patrols usually work in pairs, wearing some identifiable clothing which the children recognize. Police departments have cooperated by offering information and guidance. Shopkeepers often will cooperate by permitting use of their phones in an emergency. These patrols usually visit the schools at the beginning of the year. At that time they instruct the children to use patrolled routes and to call for help by yelling, "Police, Help" until someone assists them.

You must supplement all safety programs by knowing how your children go back and forth to school and when they can be expected to arrive home. Children must understand that strangers can be dangerous. Teach them always to tell you before going anywhere alone or with someone. Teach them to inform you about anything unusual that may occur as they go to and from school, libraries, and stores. Know who their playmates are and where they live.

School buses are being increasingly used and should be a cause for concern to all involved with child safety. Several factors have contributed to a relatively low rate of accidents involving school buses. These include the conspicuous color of school buses and the fact that these buses are generally not on the road during peak accident periods. However, these favorable conditions will be eroded as the use of buses increases. You and school supervisors must work together so that the knowledge available about vehicular safety is effectively put to use in school bussing.

Particular attention should be given to hiring physically and psychologically sound drivers who are adequately trained. Use of seat belts by drivers should be mandatory. Older buses may prove too costly to modify for greater protection. However, safety standards for new buses should include adequate padding and restraint devices to protect passengers. Information about other proven safety measures are available to both you and the educators through state highway safety organizations.

Your child must understand his contribution to bus safety. Regulations provided by schools regarding behavior on school buses are designed to maintain order and permit the driver to give full attention to driving. You have an obligation to your children to review these regulations periodically and make sure that your children are abiding by them. An adult monitor in addition to the driver may be necessary in some situations where remind-

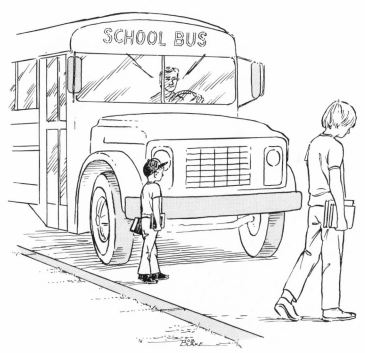

A stopped school bus discharges children and allows them to cross the road or street in front of the bus.

ers as well as rewards and punishments are insufficient to assure safe busing.

Transportation on school buses offers children special protection not available when public transportation is used. For example, a stopped school bus discharges passengers and allows them to cross the road or street in front of the bus. State laws prohibit traffic movement in either direction past the bus. Thus the bus acts as a traffic control device for the children who wish to cross. Public buses cannot do this. Young children who will use both public and school transportation need to understand the differences in the amount of protection offered against cross-traffic.

When school personnel instruct children about the dangers of running in the halls and on the playground, brief comparisons of the application of such rules between the school setting and other settings can extend the school's influence. Running in any building is generally unnecessary and inappropriate, whether it is in the home, shop-

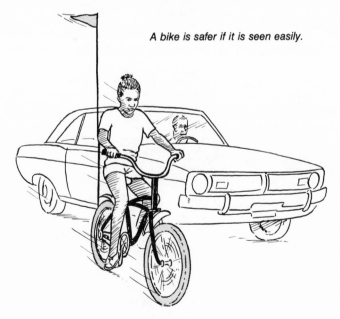

A bike is safer if it is seen easily.

ping area, or church. The reasons for restraint are the same. Schools often do more than draw comparisons about fire safety. Drills appropriate for school are not directly applicable to the home. Yet some evacuation procedure is needed at home and fire hazards must be recognized. Many schools, with the cooperation of local fire departments, provide such information and guidance.

Bicycle safety training programs offer an example of more complex school efforts to improve community and family safety patterns. Many local communities, civic organizations, and police departments are establishing bicycle safety programs. Rules of the road, proper riding techniques, and bike maintenance are included. Some schools with large numbers of children who ride bikes to school require that they pass the bike safety program before being allowed to bring bikes onto school property. The National Safety Council has available a training program for use by community groups for this purpose.

Community Recreation and Organized Sports

Playgrounds

Playground use with sophisticated and sometimes dangerous equipment has increased with population growth. You have the responsibility for knowing about such areas. You should work with recreation and municipal officials on site selection and development to assure children the greatest protection and safety. You should periodically visit and inspect the area. Appropriate and sturdy equipment plus adequate supervision are essential. Play areas should be near the center of the population to be served. Safety of children going to and from these areas should be considered. Traffic in the area should be warned of children's activities and speed limits appropriately reduced.

Equipment in playground areas should be used so as to assure partial separation of children into different groups according to age and physical maturity. All equipment must be well constructed, properly installed, and continuously maintained. Do not allow children to use defective equipment. Report such defects to an appropriate city official.

Slides should be located in shade to avoid exposing the chute to hot sun. Soft material such as sand or sawdust should be maintained at the bottom of the slide to cushion the landing. Cracks, rust, and sharp edges must be eliminated.

See-saws can smash fingers placed near the center or fulcrum of the board. Protective devices can be made part of the equipment. Children should learn, however, to keep their hands away from such areas. Two other dangerous situations can occur with see-saws: if no block is placed under the end seats, hands or feet can be caught between the board and the ground; if one rider gets off without letting the other know it, sudden elevation of one end may fling the remaining child off the raised end.

If swings are installed properly and kept in good condition, the only remaining dangers to children are then related to improper use. Standing or kneeling on swings should not be allowed. Swinging to great heights should be discouraged: children can be projected off the swing when they become frightened or let go of ropes or chains to show off. Severe injuries can occur. Do not permit an older child to swing while holding a younger one on his lap. Playing in the area of swings when they are in use should not be allowed.

Ladders, bars, and other equipment for climbing should be available in various sizes suitable for different stages of the children's development. Spaces between bars should be large enough so that heads cannot get stuck.

Sandboxes should be checked for sharp edges, broken glass, and other debris. Sandboxes are not recommended for public play areas. They are too difficult to protect from moisture as well as use and contamination by dogs and cats. Backyard sandboxes can be made small enough and covered when not in use to avoid such problems.

Wading pools should have continuously circulating water. Toddlers must be watched at all times: drowning can occur in just a few inches of water. Do not allow your child in the water if he is ill or has any skin disease or irritation.

Drinking fountains of proper height should be kept clean and free of rubbish and other debris. Teach your children to keep their mouths off the spigot and only on the stream of the water. Pushing and shoving while using fountains can result in broken teeth.

Unacceptable Areas for Play

Many hazards in your neighborhood attract children:

- Bodies of water, irrigation ditches, and excavation projects
- Underground holes or shafts from mining
- Combustible or explosive substances
- Empty houses and buildings or new construction sites
- Railroad property
- Dumps and junk yards

Children should be excluded from these areas by physical barriers. Where such barriers do not exist, exert influence on public officials to obtain this protection. In any case, help your children understand the dangers and insist that these areas not be used.

Crimeproofing Your Child

No foolproof method exists to keep your child safe from criminals. Here are some suggestions that can help:

- The old rule about never taking candy from a stranger is still valid—and the same goes for rides and even walks.
- Tell your children never to admit to being home alone, either to a phone caller or someone at the door.
- Give instructions to your child's school to release your child only in case of emergency—and only to the people you have designated in writing.
- Arrange for neighbors to help your children if an emergency occurs while you're away. Give the neighbors a phone number where you can usually be reached and offer to do the same for their children.
- If you see a child who appears lost or in trouble, be prepared to help. Don't hesitate to call the police if you think the child needs assistance.

Organized Sports Programs

Interscholastic football particularly is involved with a high percentage of sport-related injuries. For any team sport, you should be aware of at least five essentials:

- Appropriate grouping of children by weight, skill, and physical maturity
- Proper conditioning of children in preparation for actual play
- Careful coaching which considers the safety of the child with reasonable expectations for performance, for winning, and for allowing the children to have fun while competing
- Good equipment and facilities
- Adequate medical care

OTHER SIGNIFICANT HAZARDS

13

Toys, Tricycles, Bicycles

The majority of *toy*-related accidents occur for two reasons: because a toy is misused, as when a wooden block is thrown and strikes a head; because a toy is available which is unsuitable for the age of the child, as when a chemistry set is given to a six-year-old. Consumer protection laws can keep truly dangerous toys out of stores. The final responsibility rests with you who select toys. Remember the age of your child and his physical and mental development and provide supervision to assure proper use.

Playthings which are involved most frequently in serious injuries to children fall into two broad categories:

- Toys which make use of projectiles—including bows and arrows; sling shots; pea shooters; darts; air rifles; toy hand guns
- Toys that have potential for high speed accidents —including skate boards; roller skates; trikes; bikes; sleds

You can carry out your responsibilities by keeping in mind the following ideas:

1. Before buying, examine labels for age recommendations, indications that all materials are non-toxic, and Underwriter Laboratories (UL) certification of electric and fire safety.

2. Buy what suits your child's abilities and interests and

not because it is the current fad (often impressed on the child by TV programs).

3. Avoid obvious hazards of poor or fragile construction, sharp edges, and points.

4. Avoid projectile toys which can cause eye injuries and toys which produce extremely loud noises that can damage hearing.

5. After purchase, explain proper and continued safe use of the toys.

6. Continue to supervise use and play when necessary.

7. Repair broken toys or discard those which cannot be repaired.

Remember, no toy can be considered truly safe for a particular child unless the child is mentally and physically capable of using it properly. Children develop at different rates, so there is no way of setting a definite age at which a child should have a particular toy. You must make that judgment. (Remember that toys and tools handled skillfully by the twelve-year-old may cause injury to his younger brother.) The following list suggests toys suitable for children at various age levels. The list is not intended to be comprehensive; it should be used only as a general guide to the types of playthings that are safest at different ages.

Birth Up to One Year

Brightly colored objects and mobiles hung out of reach over the crib.

Rubber or washable squeak toys
Sturdy, nonflammable rattles
Washable stuffed dolls or animals

Large, brightly colored balls
Nonbreakable cups or other smooth objects to chew on

One to Two Years

Large, smooth blocks with rounded corners

Push-pull tops and wheeled animals with rounded handles

Nests of objects which fit together

Sandboxes and sturdy, rust-proof pails and shovels

or strings

Peg boards and large pegs

Small tables and chairs

Appropriate colored and illustrated books

Two to Three Years

Large blocks to fit and interlock

Wooden animals

Dolls

Sturdy kiddy cars or tricycles

Vegetable—or fruit—color finger paints

Cars and wagons to push

Miniature wheelbarrows

Modeling clay (Play-Doh)

Rocking horses

Books (appropriate)

Swing sets

Three to Six Years

Blackboards and dustless chalk

Hand puppets

Paints and paintbooks

Dollhouses and furniture

Jump ropes

Puzzle

Miniature plastic garden tools

Drums and other simple musical instruments

Phonographs and tape recorders

Books (appropriate)

Six to Eight Years

Games and puzzles

Sewing materials

Carpenter benches and tools

Construction sets

Sleds

Roller and ice skates

Kites

Playground equipment

Baseball, football, or other game balls

Puppets

Simple modeling kits

Books (appropriate)

Eight and Up

Construction and modeling kits

Electric trains, slot cars

Hand tools (hammers, planes, chisels)

Hobby equipment and materials—photography, stamp and coin collections

Games

Microscopes

Musical instruments

Chemistry sets (for eleven-year-olds and up)

Books (appropriate)

Tricycles are a special kind of toy for a special age. Most children are able to ride a trike once they have learned to go up the stairs putting one foot after the other in rotation. In addition to being able to rotate the pedals, your child must be able to follow your instructions about where and how the trike can be ridden.

Children should be taught not to ride "double." Newer trikes are being made without rear steps to discourage carrying passengers which greatly increases the trike's instability and accident potential.

Help your child understand that riding downhill is dangerous: trikes can pick up a great deal of speed very quickly and stopping safely becomes almost impossible. Sharp turns should be avoided and all turns should be made at low speeds. Do not allow your child to ride his trike down steps or curbs.

The major accident patterns associated with tricycles involve five situations:

- Poor construction of the trike which results in breakage, causing injury while in use
- Instability due to design or the trike being too large for the child
- Colliding with or striking obstacles
- Inability to stop
- Entanglement in wheels or other moving parts

You can help protect your children by purchasing well-constructed trikes which are the proper size for the individual child. Look for low-slung trikes with wheels that are widely spaced, features which improve riding stability. Choose pedals and hand grips with rough surfaces which will help prevent feet and hands from slipping.

Check the trike regularly for loose, damaged, or missing parts. Make repairs properly and get rid of sharp edges and protrusions by taping, filing down, or bending under.

Bicycles are a good source of exercise, transportation, and fun.

There are five major kinds of accidents involving bicycles:

- Loss of control
- Mechanical and/or structural problems
- Entangled feet, hands, or clothing
- Feet slipping from pedal
- Collision with another bike or with a car

You must make a careful choice about the kind of bike to purchase and then make sure it is properly ridden and taken care of. Avoid buying a bike that is too large. The child should be able to straddle the bike frame and have the horizontal bar just touch his crotch when both feet are on the ground. Seat height should be adjusted so that the child's foot remains in full contact with the pedal through the entire rotation of the pedal.

Most children under ten should have coaster brakes rather than hand brakes. *High-rise handlebars force the child to use unnatural steering techniques*. Long, narrow seats entice children to carry passengers which should not be allowed.

Proper maintenance is essential, especially of brakes, sharp edges, and worn parts. Bolts should be tightened regularly, moving parts oiled, and worn tires replaced. Complicated repairs are best done by an experienced bike mechanic.

Make sure your child's bike is equipped for the kind of riding he will do: head and tail-lights for darkness; a bag or rack to carry books that leave hands free for proper control; and close-fitting clothing with leg clips or rubber bands to keep pants from tangling with wheels, pedals, or chain. A bike is safer if it is seen easily. Use high-flying flags, reflectors, and have your child wear brightly colored clothing.

Then make sure he knows how to handle his vehicle. He must observe traffic rules, keeping to the right, signaling, traveling single file. Never allow him to "ride against traffic"—he should ride his bike always on the right side of the road. Most accidents happen at intersections, and left turns require extreme care. Walking a bike across in such situations is best. For necessary riding, help your child find alternative roads which will enable him to avoid heavy and high-speed traffic. For pleasure riding, help him choose quiet areas and bike paths which are enjoyable, interesting, and safe.

Recently young parents are riding bicycles and taking a child along. It just is not a good idea; but if you must, find out which carrier or seat is safest for your child while you ride a bicycle.

Eyeglass Safety Lenses

All children, and adults as well, who must wear eyeglasses should have safety lenses. Ninety percent of the eye injuries which occur each year in the United States could be prevented if people used protective lenses. There are two types: case-hardened glass and resin-plastic. The case-hardened lenses will not break easily and, if they do, will tend to break into small coarse granules instead of sharp slivers. The resin-plastic lenses are even safer, but are easily scratched if not handled properly. This may make them less desirable for children. Either type of safety lenses costs only slightly more than regular lenses. For growing, active children it is a necessary extra expense, particularly if they play tennis.

A hard-hit tennis ball is a dangerous object.

Protective Coloring

Children should be highly visible whenever they are in areas of traffic. This includes children who are walking and those riding bicycles. Early morning and dusk, when light is poor or there is complete darkness, are obvious times for children to be dressed in bright clothing or decorated with reflective tape. However, especially for children in rural and suburban areas, bright colors are useful at all times. Whenever children must walk or ride bikes on roadways, bright colors catch the attention of drivers quickly. The sooner a driver is aware of the child, the sooner he can adjust to prevent an accident.

Electric Shock

It is easier to prevent electric shock than it is to treat it. To a small child, an electric outlet is a fascinating hole in the wall, just right for poking. Use inexpensive and readily available childproof covers (or heavy electric tape) on unused electric outlets to keep out the baby's prying fingers and toys or other objects. Have damaged appliances and frayed cords repaired promptly. *Never let a child handle an electric cord. He may chew it.* Chewing on the "hot" end of extension cords has caused horrible mouth burns in children. Extension plugs are now available with rotary covers that prevent contact with electrically charged terminals. Old-style extension plugs should be removed if not in use or wrapped securely with electrical tape. *Do not underestimate the smallest child's capacity to tamper with electricity sources.*

You must ensure basic protection from electrical hazards throughout the house. Fuses or circuit breakers respond to electrical defects. If a fuse blows or a breaker trips, determine the cause and, if due to a wiring defect, call an electrician. Be sure to ground properly all equipment that requires it. If you are not sure what this means, ask an electrician, your fire department, or your community's office of building inspection. It is particularly important to ground TV sets, power tools, and any equipment near grounded objects such as water pipes.

Use extension and appliance cords that are heavy enough to carry the amount of current required. Do not use lamp cords for heating appliances. Do not use electrical appliances where they can get wet. Home electrical repairs should be done by experienced individuals. Change light bulbs with lamp or fixture disconnected. Follow all instructions supplied with the electrical equipment you buy.

Remember that shock hazards are greatest in bathrooms, kitchens, and basements, and around water.

Wringer Safety

There are still thousands of clothes-wringer accidents per year in the United States. The washing machine with a wringer is not out of use, particularly in isolated and rural areas, and thousands are sold annually. The Underwriters' Laboratories have adopted new safety standards in an effort to reduce wringer injuries to children. These standards require that power to the wringer be controlled by the operator or that the rollers stop turning if force is applied opposite to the direction of the infeed.

Follow the recommendations listed below:

1. When children are around, and you must leave the washer—even for a moment—turn the switch off and pull the electric plug from the outlet.

2. Check the wringer's safety release. Test the release each time you start washing. Be sure it works properly,

and practice releasing it until your action will be instinctive in case of an accident. Every member of the family old enough to understand should be familiar with that release mechanism. Use the safety release in case of an accident. Do not reverse the rollers.

3. Keep children away from the washer. It is not a toy, and the wringer can be dangerous. Warn the children to stay away from it and never let them play with it or operate it.

4. If a hand or arm is caught between the rollers of the wringer, remember that this is a crush injury, the seriousness of which may not be immediately apparent. See your physician without delay.

Animals

Pets

Family pets can be fun for children, as well as for all of the family. You should realize, however, that toddlers and children under five are apt to abuse pets. While it is possible for children to get certain type of dog worm infections and cat scratch disease, frequently the young child is more of a hazard to the pet than the pet to the child. When purchasing a family pet, consider the maturity and disposition of both your child and the animal. Make certain your child is not allergic to the animal. Have your pets properly immunized against rabies, distemper, infectious hepatitis, and leptospirosis.

Caution your child not to disturb a sleeping animal, tease it, overexcite it in play, make threatening gestures toward it, or remove its food. Play should be gentle.

When dogs run in a pack, they may become vicious. Teach your children to be cautious with dogs, even your own, when they are in a group.

Children should learn to participate in the proper care and feeding of pets. Food and water should be provided under conditions safe for the child. For example, if a dog has been confined for several hours it may become highly excited by the smell of food or the approach of any person. Parents should establish patterns of care which allow animals reasonable freedom, with confinement in appropriate space. If fenced areas are not available, dogs should be tied in ways which allow some movement and exercise without entanglement. An affectionate and cooperative animal can be changed into a mean and obstinate one by inappropriate care. Dogs should be leashed when being walked.

Remember that the small child will put anything in his mouth. Keep your child away from places where dog droppings might exist. Also keep your dog clean by washing with soap and water his entire body. Your child will have his mouth all over the pet when he is playing with it. Serious worm infections can result.

Help your child make friends with animals he will frequently meet in your neighborhood and on his way to school. Teach him not to be afraid of other people's pets, but to use caution in making friends with them. He should not make the first move towards friendship and *never* hold his face close to an animal's mouth. Let the animal make the first friendly move after it sniffs the child.

Tell your child never to remove a pup from his mother's attention. Even the most gentle female dog will react, sometimes violently.

Strange Domestic Animals

Teach your child to ignore strange dogs. In addition, for his protection he should learn how to deal with dogs that cannot be ignored. Your child should learn to avoid routes where animals chase cars, bicycles, or tricycles. Teach him to drop immediately any food he is eating when approached by an animal. Never allow your child to stop an animal fight or go near or try to pet strange, sick, injured, wild, or nervous animals.

Tell your child that if he is carrying something, to tuck it under his arm: the swinging motion of his hand and the object may excite the animal.

If the dog growls or seems to want to bite, instruct your child to stand perfectly still, to keep his hands at his sides, and to avoid looking the dog in the eye. Usually the dog will lose interest and go away.

If the dog does not go away, suggest to your child that he begin talking to it in a soothing manner. When the dog seems to have accepted him, he should walk toward the dog, past it and away. Tell your child: *Never move quickly or to run. Do not pet the dog.*

If a dog attacks without warning, instruct your child to fold his arms, grabbing each elbow with the opposite hand, and thrust his arms up in front of his face. If the dog knocks him down, he should roll onto his stomach and protect his head and neck with his arms. Then he should lie absolutely still.

Wild Animals

Animals confined in zoos of various kinds will not harm your children if you see to it that the children behave appropriately. Instructions to visitors should be followed. If feeding is not allowed, *do not feed*. Fences and cages are for mutual protection. Fingers and arms poked through enclosures provoke caged animals and can result in severe injury.

When traveling in national parks or other areas where wild animals are likely to be encountered, avoid direct contact with all animals, large or small. Ordinarily, animals in the wild will not approach people but rather run away. Bites and other injuries occur when people try to capture or simply touch the animals; then the animal will feel trapped and is very likely to fight back in the only way he knows. Look and admire, but keep your distance.

Christmas time

Most accidents at Christmas time happen because of unsafe or improper use of decorations, particularly those that have electrical connections. Candles, trees, and fireplaces also represent hazards.

Christmas trees that are natural should be fresh. Test this by tapping the base of the tree against the ground. If many needles fall off you have a dry tree. Keep the tree outside as long as possible, preferably with the base of the trunk in a pail of water—not ice. Once indoors the tree should stand in a stable base which contains water. Avoid placing trees near heat sources of any kind. It is almost impossible to flameproof trees completely at home. Therefore do not use lighted candles on trees or near any other evergreen decorations. Dispose of the natural tree when needles begin to fall. Anchoring the back of the tree with a sturdy string or insulated wire to a baseboard or wall is good protection from children pulling the tree down.

Metal trees can be a source of severe shock when electric lights are attached. Colored floodlights or spotlights are the only safe way to illuminate a metal tree. These lamps become very hot and should be positioned out of reach of children.

Plastic trees should be made of fire-resistant materials —which means they will not catch fire easily. *There are no completely fireproof plastic trees.*

Impress on your small child that he should look but not touch the Christmas tree once it is decorated. Trees not well based can be pulled down by clutching little fingers. To satisfy his excitement, help him place decorations on the tree (never without your presence).

All lights should bear the UL label of Underwriters Laboratories. Check older equipment for frayed and exposed wires, loose connections, and broken sockets. Repair or discard unsafe equipment. Bulbs should not be in contact with needles or decorations. Outdoor lights should be waterproof and clearly marked for outdoor

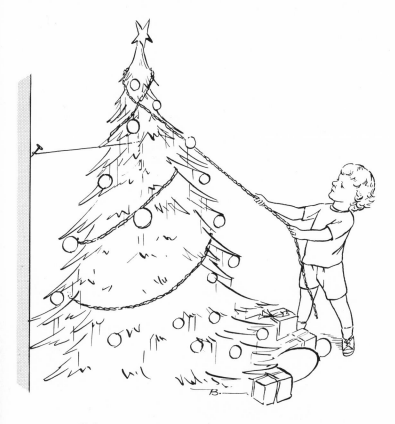

Christmas trees not well-based can be pulled down by little clutching fingers.

use. *Always disconnect from the wall outlet* all lights when you go to bed or leave the house.

Fireplaces should be used only with screens in place and well anchored. Do not burn large quantities of wrapping paper, boxes or evergreen branches in the fireplace at one time; they may throw sparks and burning scraps into the room.

Children may eat several kinds of Christmas items that may be poisonous. These include: holly and mistletoe berries, fire salts, tinsel containing lead. Children also are often cut by broken ornaments.

Review your fire safety plans with your family. Fires at Christmas-time are the source of many deaths and disabling injuries.

Halloween

The greatest dangers to children at Halloween are from accidents in traffic and injuries related to costumes and masks. Costumes should be bright and decorated with reflective tape. They should be made of flame-retardant fabric, short enough to avoid tripping. Masks should not interfere with seeing or breathing. Plastic bags should never be used, even if holes are cut. A "mask" applied directly to the skin and made with cosmetics is the safest.

Children should not carry candles, even inside a pumpkin.

You should do the following to protect trick-or-treaters:

- Stay in your own neighborhood where the children are known and recognized.
- Accompany small children, day or night.
- Check all treats before allowing the children to eat anything they receive.

- Remind children of traffic safety rules.
- Tell children to avoid poorly lighted areas and to stay out no more than two hours after dusk.

Fireworks

Blindings, severe burns, amputations, and deaths occur when fireworks are used carelessly. *Children do not understand the dangers of fireworks.* The Federal Government has prohibited the sale to the general public of the most dangerous kinds of fireworks. But fireworks including dangerous ones continue to be available in some states. Injuries and deaths continue to occur often even when so-called "safe" fireworks are used. For example, sparklers burn at extremely high temperatures. Clothing can

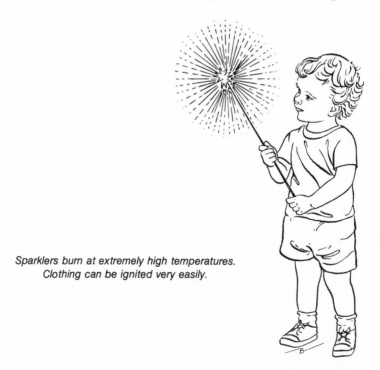

Sparklers burn at extremely high temperatures. Clothing can be ignited very easily.

be ignited very easily. Young children should not be allowed to use fireworks under any circumstances. Older children should use fireworks only with adult supervision.

Babysitters and Child-care Workers in the Home

The person who cares for your children in your absence should be capable of maintaining safety and protection for them. Only individuals who have a sense of responsibility and are old enough and capable enough to assume that responsibility should be entrusted with your children. You can find sitters by asking friends and relatives for those whom they have found to be reliable. Various community organizations such as Y's, scouts, high schools, colleges, and church groups can recommend individuals and fee schedules.

Once a sitter is chosen, you should satisfy yourself that the individual can measure up to your expectations. Personal cleanliness and good physical health and mental attitude are essential. Attitudes about children should be friendly and result in cooperation and enjoyment with the child. You should find out how much the sitter understands about the specific care your child will need such as feeding infants, restricting toddlers, and maintaining good discipline with older children.

It is your responsibility to provide sufficient information for the sitter to use. Be sure to introduce the sitter to your child. If the child is sleeping, show the sitter where the child is. Tell your sitter specifically what you want done. Demonstrate any procedure with which your sitter may not be familiar. *Do not allow a sitter to give your baby a tub bath:* instruct the sitter to do any necessary washing with a face cloth.

Give the sitter information about your children's peculiar habits, about hazards that attract them, and how you can be reached by phone. If your children are not to be permitted to do something during your absence which they ordinarily might do when you are home, tell the children in the presence of the sitter.

Give the sitter specific instructions for dealing with emergencies:

In case of fire or smoke

Get the children out immediately, without stopping to dress them or to make a phone call. Take the children to the nearest neighbor: Then call the Fire Department first, you (the parents) second.

In case of sudden illness

Have a phone number available to call for assistance, either where you will be, a substitute adult in a position to make a decision about what to do, or the family doctor.

In case of serious injury

Agree on what is serious injury. Plan to use your community's most efficient source of emergency care such as Rescue Squad or Police Department for transportation to a hospital emergency room. **Call the source of emergency care first, you (the parents) second.** Explain what is wrong and who has been called.

If there are pets, the sitter should be comfortable with them. Jealous dogs and other pets with which the sitter is not at ease should be confined in ways acceptable to the sitter.

Agree on certain behavior which if observed routinely by the sitter offers additional assurance of safe care:

• Do not open the door to strangers.

- Never leave the children alone in the house even for a minute.
- Do not invite or allow friends into the home (unless the sitter has obtained your prior consent).
- Stay alert and absorbed in working with the children: do not be distracted by personal telephone calls, blaring radio or records, or television.

Similarly, parents should agree to behave in certain ways: allow enough time between the arrival of a sitter and your departure to discuss all arrangements; return on time or call if unavoidably delayed.

When Adults Put Children in Danger

Adults unintentionally put children in danger under certain circumstances. Most accidents occur when normal, healthy people are experiencing four specific kinds of stress or circumstance:

- When they become ill or injured.
- When they are unusually fatigued.
- When they have been drinking alcoholic beverages to excess.
- When they are experiencing difficult personal problems.

During such stressful times adults are distracted easily from thinking about safety. Physical discomfort, irritability, impatience, uncomfortable thoughts compete for attention. Late for work and school, the children pile in the car and the seat belts are forgotten; impatience and distractions at an intersection lead to a collision. A sequence of thoughtless and hurried events results in an accident.

The terms "emotional strain" and "conflict" are often used to describe feelings and behavior of people involved in various kinds of accidents. Both happy and sad events can contribute to such strain and conflict. Such occassions are part of everyone's life. Recognizing these times of stress and considering some of them in advance may help prepare you for dealing with them when they occur.

There are times and events that are known to be associated with stress and with higher than normal accident potential. Some of these are:

Physical status and health

This includes temporary abnormal circumstances such as severe colds or flu; normal physical changes such as pregnancy and menstruation; hospitalization; permanent changes in physical condition such as a new diagnosis of diabetes in a parent.

Emotional stress

This includes death of a family member; separation or divorce; problems at work; tense relationships between parents.

Family life changes

This includes moving to a new residence or community; changing schools; loss of job; changes in financial status or needs; addition of a new family member through, for example, birth of a child; grandparents moving in.

There are many other times and events in our lives which will cause stress. Think about yourself and the people around you. Try to recognize when you may be most susceptible to the effects of stress. Adjust your activities and your behavior to adapt to these difficult occasions. Be especially aware of safety problems and how to cope with them.

HAZARDS
(OVERVIEW)

14

General, or Generic, Hazards*

Many hazards, such as electrical shock, high surface temperatures, sharp edges, or poisonous chemicals, appear among a broad range of products. These hazards can be divided into four general or generic categories: (1) thermal (or heat), (2) electrical, (3) mechanical, and (4) chemical. Awareness of these generic hazards in your home can help to prevent accidents and injuries:

Thermal (Heat) Hazards

Thermal, or heat, hazards can develop from fire and heat sources. Some of the hazards are obvious, such as getting clothing too close to the flame of a gas stove or dropping a match or lighted cigarette on nightclothes or bedding. But others may not be so obvious, such as flammable vapors from gasoline being ignited by a distant pilot light in a gas water heater. Hot cooking utensils can burn a child, and even hot water in a bathtub can cause burns.

Electrical Hazards

Electrical fire can develop when circuits are overloaded (when too much current flows through wiring). Electrical

* This chapter is reprinted with minor and nonsubstantive editing from "Technical Fact Sheet," U.S. Consumer Product Safety Commission, Washington, D.C., with the approval of the Commission.

shock can develop when current flows through your child's body (because of a short circuit or an appliance malfunction). The most common injuries resulting from accidents involving electrical hazards are burns and shock, both of which can have lasting, damaging effects on your child.

Mechanical Hazards

Mechanical hazards can develop from sharp edges, sharp points, poorly balanced products (such as some high chairs), and slippery walking surfaces. These hazards may be the most universal since almost every product can cause you to fall or cut yourself. The most common injuries resulting from accidents involving mechanical hazards are cuts, bruises, and broken bones. Some of these may be relatively minor, such as stubbing a toe on a bed post or spraining an ankle when your child trips on the stairs. But some accidents involving mechanical hazards can result in death. The most frequent cause of accidental death in the U.S. is auto accidents, but the second most frequent cause of accidental death is falls, often resulting from mechanical hazards in and around the home.

Chemical Hazards

Certain household products such as cleaners, bleaches, flammable solvents, insecticides, drugs, and paints contain ingredients which may present chemical hazards if the directions for use are not followed or if they are intentionally misused. These products may be toxic if swallowed, breathed, or absorbed. They may be corrosive or irritant to eyes or skin. In addition, some of these products may be flammable or create pressure through heat or other means. The ingredients present in an aerosol may contribute to a chemical hazard if the directions for use are not followed. Carbon monoxide produced by fuel-burning appliances may present a chemical hazard, particularly if these appliances are used in a room without sufficient fresh air.

Overview

Here are some products which are associated with these generic hazards. Remember: there may be more than one hazard associated with some products.

Thermal (Heat) Hazards

Kitchen ranges and ovens
Space heaters and radiators
Fireplaces
Flammable fabrics

Flammable liquids
Counter-top cooking appliances
Hot water in the bathroom, kitchen, or other rooms
Irons

Electrical Hazards

Electric hair dryers, toasters, refrigerators, and other appliances
House wiring

Electric saws, drills, and other tools
Extension cords and wall sockets

Mechanical Hazards

Power lawn mowers, power saws, and other cutting machines
Glass doors, walls, and windows
Glass bottles
Ladders

Children's furniture (cribs, high chairs, infant seats)
Wringer washing machines
Playground equipment
Toys
Bicycles
Stairs

Chemical Hazards

Drugs, household cleaners, bleaches, and flammable liquids
Insectides and pesticides

Fuel-burning appliances, which produce carbon monoxide
Aerosols

Safety tips for specific products are available free from the U.S. Consumer Product Safety Commission, but there are many suggestions for dealing with generic hazards. Your home will be safer if you can answer "Yes" to all of the questions in the following checklist:

Thermal (Heat) Hazards

☐ Do space heaters, fireplaces, and other heat sources have guards so that you can't touch the flames or heating elements?

☐ Are drapes and furniture away from gas and electric ranges and baseboard heaters which could ignite them?

☐ Are matches and lighters kept out of reach of children?

☐ Are flammable liquids stored and used away from pilot lights?

☐ Are pot handles turned toward the back of the stove so that a child won't spill the hot food onto himself?

☐ Do you stay with pre-school children when they are near hot water in the bathtub?

☐ Do you have proper fire-extinguisher and smoke-alarm equipment?

Electrical Hazards

☐ Are grounding type 3-wire electrical appliances properly grounded? (top, single hole in outlet usually is ground.)

☐ Are electrical appliances out of the bathroom so that you or your child won't touch them while wet?

☐ Are extension cords, outlets, and circuits not overloaded?

☐ Do you know how to disconnect the main switch in your electric switchbox in an emergency?

☐ Are electric cords out of reach so they can't be pulled or tripped over?

□ Do unused outlets have dummy plugs to keep children from getting shocked?

□ Are appliance cords and extension cords in good repair and neatly tucked away from toddler's hands?

Mechanical Hazards

□ Are glass doors and walls marked with decals so that people can see them from both directions? Is safety glass used?

□ Are drinking glasses used by children unbreakable?

□ Are lawn mowers and other cutting machines in good repair, with all necessary guards?

□ Are there no small rugs near stairs? Is there a gate at the top of stairs to prevent small children from falling?

□ Are there handrails along the wall down the stairs?

□ Is all children's furniture stable and free of sharp edges?

□ Are children's toys free of sharp edges, small parts, and breakable or removable parts?

□ Are bicycles, playground equipment, and other recreational equipment free of protrusions, sharp edges, and other parts which could cut or bruise?

Chemical Hazards

□ Have you read the *label* of the household agent before purchasing?

□ Are all household chemical products locked up away from children?

□ Are those products which have safety packaging properly closed?

□ Are all household substances that are purchased in bulk (such as gasoline), or which have been transferred from their original containers, kept in sturdy, clearly labeled, non-food containers?

☐ Are your gas appliances checked annually to insure that they are not releasing deadly carbon monoxide into the home?

If you find a product hazard or a product-related injury, write to the U.S. Consumer Product Safety Commission, Washington, D. C. 20207. In the continental United States, call the toll-free hotline: 800-638-2666.

PART FOUR

Care and Treatment After Injury

INTRODUCTION

Information about care and treatment after injury is intended to enable you and your older children to act responsibly when injury to your child occurs, particularly in the home environment. Accidents are threatening and unpleasant even for those not injured. Proper preparation for emergencies can prevent panic on the part of not only the injured child but also those attempting to offer help. Action can then be taken with confidence to provide immediate temporary care to save a life, reduce disability, and improve chances for full recovery.

Here we shall provide some principles of first aid about common situations with adequate but simple and sensible measures that can be used effectively and immediately in and about the home or at the site where the injury occurs. More intensive training in first aid is readily available throughout the United States from the American National Red Cross programs.

Accidents always strike unexpectedly, and the person who may be called upon to render first aid should have up-to-date knowledge available for quick action. You should become thoroughly familiar with the home first aid charts in this book (for accidents and poisoning) since they are basic, useful, and easily accessible. (These are printed beginning on page 289.) Always take this book along when you travel for any period of time with your children, particularly in remote areas.

Three categories of injury and treatment will be reviewed in this section:

1. *Life-threatening situations.*
2. *Dangerous medical situations.*
3. *Minor medical situations.*

These categories allow us to group accidents or situations leading to injury as they are experienced most commonly. Suggestions will be offered about how a given injury should be dealt with at the beginning. Any given accident or situation may be different, and when you give help to your child, you must decide quickly how urgent is the need for additional medical care.

LIFE-THREATENING SITUATIONS

15

In this chapter the basic life-saving techniques that you may be called upon to use in some life-threatening situations will be presented. These techniques include:

- Artificial respiration (rescue breathing)
- Controlling severe bleeding
- Treating injury-related shock
- Cardiopulmonary resuscitation

The life-threatening situations include:

- Poisonings
- Breathing failure and choking:
    in drowning
    electric shock
    obstruction in airway (windpipe)
- Extensive burns

General Guidelines

Some general guidelines should be observed when dealing with any of the life-threatening situations. As soon as you realize first aid must be given, call for professional help immediately or, better still, have someone else call while you administer first aid. The most accessible professional assistance should be obtained. This will vary from community to community. Make immediate use of your rescue squad, police or fire departments, or physician. Do not waste time searching for telephone numbers. Dial the Operator, give your address, a brief description of the emergency situation, and request emergency help. Some communities have a short emergency telephone number. Keep it displayed for instant use. Be sure that your house number is quickly visible from the street, particularly at night. Turn on all outside lights your dwelling may have.

Always assume all accident victims are alive unless *very* obvious signs are present to indicate the contrary. One person (if it is you, don't hesitate to take the responsibility) should take charge of dealing with the emergency. You should enlist help from bystanders, but you must remain in control of the situation.

While you are waiting for professional help to arrive, first aid care should follow these priorities:

- Remove the victim from any source of continuing danger such as fire, smoke, electric current, water.
- Make sure the victim can breathe (clear the airway, or windpipe, if needed).
- Control severe bleeding.
- Prevent, if you can, injury-related shock.

You must know how to administer artificial respiration (rescue breathing) and to control bleeding in order to deal with these priorities. Here we will outline these techniques as well as ways for preventing injury-related shock. In the information which follows we will mention only the necessity for using these techniques rather than repeat them each time. It is important, then, for you to learn these techniques and practice them in "dry-run" or make-believe situations so that they become automatic. Practice them with your oldest child (over fourteen) as the "victim"; he will also learn from the experience.

Artificial Respiration—the Rescue Breathing Technique

1. Place your child on his back.

2. Clear the throat. Turn your child's head to one side, force his mouth open if necessary, and wipe out with your fingers any fluid, vomitus, mucus, or foreign body.

3. With his head now face up, tilt his head backward. Extend the neck as far as possible. This will automatically keep the tongue out of the airway.

4. Blow—with your baby's lips closed, breathe into his nose with a smooth, steady action until his chest is seen to rise. Stop breathing into the nostrils and allow lungs to expel the forced air. For older children, use the mouth-to-mouth technique. (The mouth-to-mouth technique is described below under *Cardiopulmonary Resuscitation.*)

5. Repeat—continue with relatively shallow breaths (appropriate for your child's size) at the rate of about 15-20 breaths per minute. For infants, only small puffs should be used.

If you are not getting air exchange, quickly recheck the position of his head, turn the child on his side, and give several sharp blows between the shoulder blades to jar foreign matter free that may be in his windpipe. Sweep fingers through your child's mouth and throat again to remove foreign matter. **Do not stop.** If his chest can be observed to rise and fall, all within your power is being done correctly for the moment.

Cardiopulmonary Resuscitation

This technique is used when there is cardiac (or heart) arrest and should be done by trained people *if they are available immediately.* If they are not, until qualified help arrives, you must do something to:

- Relieve airway obstruction (clear the throat, or windpipe, of any lodged materials).
- Restore breathing.
- Restore circulation.

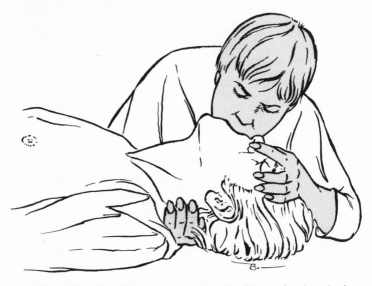

Rapidly ventilate the child's lungs by giving him three or four breaths (a breath per second) mouth-to-mouth. (In infants, breaths through the nostrils may be easier and more effective, in which case keep the mouth closed.)

The child should be placed on his back, preferably on a firm support such as the floor, a table, or a bed board. Make sure his airway is open by wiping out his mouth and throat, free of all obstructions. Rapidly ventilate the child's lungs by giving him three or four deep breaths (a breath per second), mouth-to-mouth. In small children and infants, breaths through the nostrils may be easier and more effective. Give a sharp blow to the heart area; this alone may restore heart activity. If it does not, place the heel of one hand in the center of the chest over the

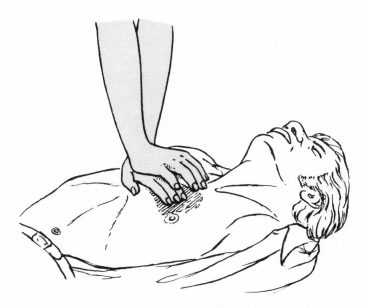

If blowing air into the child's mouth and a sharp blow to the heart area do
not restore heart activity, place the heel of one hand in the center of
the chest and the other hand on top of it. (For infants, use
your fingers as shown in the bottom illustration.) Exert
pressure as described in the accompanying text.

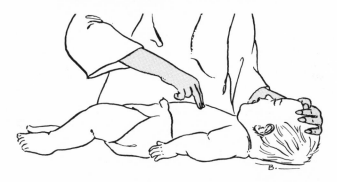

lower portion of the breastbone and place the other hand
on top of it. Rock forward and use the weight of your
body (not fully for infants and young children) to exert
pressure downward. Now lift your weight. Repeat this
rhythmic compression approximately fifteen times. Each
time you bear down, you squeeze the child's heart, forc-

ing blood out to his body, actually substituting for his heartbeat. After about a minute or a minute and a half, or 15 compressions, stop the massage and fill his lungs again with fresh air. If there is someone else present, have him ventilate the lungs simultaneously. There is no need to synchronize the two lifesaving procedures.

In infants the breastbone should be depressed with the fingers. Excessive pressure should be avoided.

Controlling Severe Bleeding

Have your child lie down. To stop bleeding, press a sterile dressing—or a clean handkerchief or the cleanest cloth item at hand (shirt-tail, etc.)—firmly over the wound. If the dressing becomes saturated with blood, lay a fresh dressing directly over the saturated one and continue pressure. As a last resort, press your hand over the wound.

If direct pressure doesn't work, pressure *both above and below* the wound often will stop the bleeding. Or try shutting off circulation in the artery supplying the blood to the wound by pressing firmly against it with your hand or fingers. There are four points (see illustration) where arterial pressure is practical for those giving first-aid. But don't try arterial pressure for wounds of the head, neck, and trunk.

Bandage the wound firmly after bleeding stops. Treatment and cleaning of the wound should be done by a physician.

Treating Shock Due to Injury

Shock occurs with any serious injury (such as a bleeding wound, a fracture, or severe burns), and good and

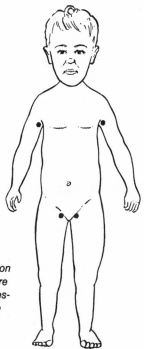

If severe bleeding occurs, and direct pressure on the wound will not stop the bleeding, then there are four pressure points on the body where pressure may control arterial bleeding. Be sure to read the text for precautions.

adequate first aid could be the most important part of treatment.

Symptoms: The skin is pale, cold, and clammy; the pulse is rapid; breathing is shallow (short) or irregular; and the injured child is frightened, restless, and apprehensive.

Treatment: Keep your child lying down, face up. Keep his airway open. If he vomits, turn his head to one side so that his neck is arched. Elevate his legs *if there are no broken bones.* Keep your child warm, but not overly so, and give him shock fluid (1 teaspoonful of salt, 1½ teaspoonsful baking soda in one quart water) *if he is able to swallow* (never give liquids to an unconscious person). *Reassure him* (this is important).

Shock should not be confused with simple *fainting*. Individuals with minor injuries may faint simply from the sight of blood or a gaping wound. A child who has fainted looks pale and is often covered with perspiration; the pulse usually will be slow rather than rapid as in shock, and recovery will occur promptly if he is allowed to lie flat with his feet elevated. If your child cannot be moved from a sitting position, lower the head between the knees.

Poisonings

Whenever your child has swallowed any poison, the principle of first aid is to get the poison out or dilute it. Call for professional help immediately: your doctor, poison control center, pharmacy, hospital, police, or fire department. Tell them what has been swallowed and follow their instructions. If you cannot obtain help immediately and must begin first aid, you must choose the proper first aid measure that is best for the situation you have. (See also Chapter 6.)

If your child is unconscious or in convulsions, do not try to induce vomiting or dilute the poison by forcing liquids. Make sure your child can breathe. Administer artificial respiration if necessary. Keep your child warm and transport him to the hospital immediately. Try to obtain the container of the poison he swallowed and any remaining contents, as well as any vomited material. This will help the doctor in rapid identification of the poison so that proper treatment can be started quickly.

If you do not know what your child has swallowed and he is conscious, do not induce vomiting. Dilute the poison with water or milk by forcing fluids into your child's mouth. Take your child to the hospital immediately. Take the poison container, if it is easily available, or any vomitus with you.

If you know that your child has swallowed a poison that is **not** *a strong acid, strong alkali, or petroleum product,* dilute the poison with water or milk by forcing the fluids into your child's mouth. Petroleum products include gasoline, kerosene, furniture polish, naphtha, charcoal lighter fluid, mineral spirits (benzine), paint thinner, Stoddard solvent. Strong acids include toilet bowl cleaners, rust removers. Strong alkalis include household bleach, drain cleaners, washing soda. Use one to two cups of water or milk for children under five years and up to one quart of water for children five years and older. *Do not use carbonated beverages,* e.g., soda pop, etc. Induce vomiting for all ingested poisons except for caustic acids or alkalis and petroleum products, or if the child is stuporous or unconscious.

To induce vomiting:

- Give one tablespoon (½ ounce) of syrup of ipecac for a child one year of age or older (under one year of age, give two teaspoons) plus at least one cup of water.
- If no ipecac syrup is available, tickle back of throat with a spoon handle or other blunt object, after giving water. *Do not give salt or mustard to children in case of poisoning.* Table salt can be dangerous and mustard is usually ineffective.
- If no vomiting occurs in 20 minutes, this ipecac dose may be repeated *once only.* In infants, vomiting is often expedited by agitation (mixing the stomach contents by gentle shaking of the infant). After vomiting has ceased, offer a mixture of activated charcoal (1-2 tablespoonsful) in a glass of water. Activated charcoal is black and gritty and it is difficult to get children to take the mixture. The addition of chocolate or other syrup, if available, can be a great help in this regard.
- If no vomiting occurs, do not waste time waiting.

Telephone (doctor, poison control center, hospital, police or fire department) for further instructions, or transport your child to a medical facility. Bring container of the poison with you.

- If vomiting does occur, keep your child's head face down to avoid choking. A small child can be placed face down across your knees.

Breathing Failure and Choking

Breathing failure can occur because of numerous causes such as drowning, electric shock, or choking on food or objects which shut off the child's airway (windpipe). The rescue and treatment techniques for a given situation have their own specific characteristics.

Drowning

Rescue. Get the child out of the water as quickly as possible. Remember three words: *Throw, Row, Go*. First, THROW. Throw a life preserver to him or swim toward him with one; or push a large plank toward him or any other floating object that will support his weight. Second, ROW. If a boat is available, go to your child immediately and render assistance, being careful that in his fright he doesn't pull you into the water. Third, GO. Swim to him only as a last resort, when other means of rescue are not available. The swimming rescue of an actively drowning person is difficult and dangerous; it is best undertaken by someone trained in lifesaving.

Treatment. Do not carry your drowning child any farther than absolutely necessary after you have removed him from the water. Lay him down quickly on his face. *Start artificial respiration at once* if breathing has stopped or if it is irregular. Don't delay for any reason—seconds can mean the difference between a life saved and a life lost.

Water in the lungs cannot be "poured out," and valuable time should not be lost in trying to empty anything but the upper air passages.

Frequently the stomach of a drowning person is greatly distended with swallowed water following submersion. In such cases, after resuscitation has been started, it is helpful to place your hands under your child's waist and lift. This tends to compress and empty the stomach, which facilitates breathing, circulation, and recovery. Send for medical aid promptly.

Choking on Food or Other Objects

When your child's airway (windpipe) is blocked, you have about four or five minutes to save his life.

A person who is choking can be distinguished from one having a heart attack or other medical problem. Usually children are not subject to heart attacks. However, to be sure, quickly ask your child to move his head and to speak. His ability to understand you indicates that he is conscious, but if he is unable to speak you must assume his airway is blocked.

Stand behind your child and put both arms around his waist. Let his head, arms, and upper body hang forward. Grasp your fist with your other hand and place it against your child's stomach slightly above the navel at the waist-line. Press your fist up rapidly against your child's stomach, repeating several times until the food or other object pops out. (This technique is called the *Heimlich maneuver*.)

If your child is too large for you to hold, have him lie on his back. Kneel over the child and press crossed hands firmly against his stomach just above the waist-line. A second person should be ready to reach firmly and remove with his fingers the ejected food or object from the child's mouth.

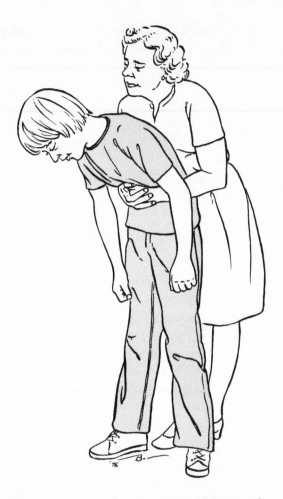

*Press your fist up rapidly against your child's stomach,
repeating several times until the food or other
object pops out.*

Continued difficulty in breathing after food has been
removed may require artificial respiration.

It is possible for an older child himself to use a variation of this technique to expel the object. Teach him the
technique. He should press his fist against his stomach
just above the waistline or press against the back of a
chair, the edge of a sink, counter or table.

Any child who has experienced airway, or windpipe, blockage should be examined further by a physician.

Burns

In the care and treatment of burns you should avoid contamination of the injured areas, relieve the pain, and prevent shock. In the case of scalding water, remove the clothing as quickly as possible. All children experiencing major burns should be checked for breathing difficulty. If necessary, begin artifical respiration promptly. *Never apply vaseline, butter, lard, cold cream, antiseptics, or any other substance on a serious burn. This can cause infection and further injury. Do not put cotton on any burn.*

Degree and Extensiveness of Burns

There are three degrees of burns:

1. **First-degree burns.** Reddening of the skin but no damage to the deeper layers of the skin structure.

2. **Second-degree burns.** Blistering of the skin as the result of injury to the deeper skin layers, but there is no damage to the structures beneath.

3. **Third-degree burns.** Charred or "cooked" appearance. The skin is burned off or severely damaged, and the underlying structures are injured.

Extensiveness of the burn. The seriousness of a burn is determined not only by the degree of its severity but also by the *extent* of its area. For example, a *second-degree burn* covering a large area like the chest is likely to be more serious than a *third-degree burn* involving only a small part of the body such as a finger. Even second or third-degree burns involving 10 percent or more of the total body are serious. Burns of this extent are likely to cause shock and can result in later complications.

Burns in children are, in general, more serious than burns of the same severity and extensiveness in adults. The amount of surface area involved can be calculated by the so-called "rule of 9's." These figures will aid in determining the prognosis of the burned individual. Each of the following areas represents 9 percent: the *head and neck*, *each upper extremity* (or arms), the *front chest*, the *back chest*, the *abdomen*, the *back*, the *front half of each lower extremity* (or legs), and the *back half of each lower extremity*; the *genitalia* are considered 1 percent.

Heat Burns (from fire, hot liquids, etc.)

Lay the injured child down gently with his head slightly lower than the rest of his body. Don't remove any more clothing than is necessary to get at the burned area, but do remove any clothing containing scalding water. If *clothing sticks* to the burned area, don't attempt to pull it off. Cut around it with scissors, and leave it on the burned area. Bacterial infection of burned areas is to be avoided. Do not touch the burned area with hands or clothing. Cover your nose and mouth with a mask if available while examining the burn and while applying a protective dressing to it. (This will help keep any germs in your nose, throat, and mouth from contaminating the burned area and increasing the hazard of infection.) A satisfactory mask can be made from a clean handkerchief, a clean cloth folded several times, or several thicknesses of gauze bandage.

Cover the burned area completely with sterile, *dry* gauze bandage. If sterile gauze is not available, use clean cloth, preferably a non-cotton towel, pillowcase, or sheet. Use material which has been recently washed, unused, and ironed; carefully unfold it so that an inside, untouched surface is applied against the burn. Do not tape bandage on so tightly that it cuts off circulation, but make it snug enough to protect the burned area from the air. If enough material is available, make the bandage thick.

Another method is to submerge the burned area in cold water (under 70°F.) and keep adding ice to maintain the temperature. (This is ideal treatment for localized minor, painful burns.) Parts of the body that cannot be submerged should be treated with a non-sticking cloth that has been dipped in cold water. Treatment should continue until the burned parts can be kept out of the cold water without recurrence of pain.

Treat for shock; if the burned child is conscious and does not have accompanying abdominal injury, give shock solution by mouth (1 teaspoonful of salt and one and one-half teaspoonful baking soda, diluted in one quart of water). Keep the child lying down. Cover him with blankets or other covers for warmth, but do not cause overheating and sweating. Move the burned child with special care. Get him to professional medical help as soon as possible.

Chemical Burns

Burns produced by strong chemicals, such as battery fluid or other acids, lye, or other strong alkalis, should be flushed off immediately with plenty of water. Hold the burned area under the cold-water faucet or pour cold water over the area. While flushing the area with water, *remove* any clothing that may be soaked with the chemical. Continue flushing the burned area with cold water until all the chemical has been washed away. For strong alkali burns of the skin, a bandage soaked with a solution of vinegar diluted one-half with water can be effectively applied. Then proceed as directed for heat burns.

Chemical Burns of the Eye. Burns of the eye from lye, lime, battery fluid, and other chemicals can cause serious damage to vision. Eyelids must be opened and, because of pain, may have to be held open.

Flush the eye immediately with large amounts of cool water. This can be done by turning the head over and holding it under the stream from a cold-water faucet if such a faucet is readily available. The stream of water should be sufficiently heavy to flush out the chemical but not so forceful that it will damage the eye. Another method is to hold the eye over the stream of water from a drinking fountain.

Promptness is of great importance; do not take your injured child any great distance to a faucet or drinking fountain if any other source of cool, clean water is available. Have your child lie down with the head tilted slightly backward. Gently pour water into his eye from a container such as a glass, cup, or pitcher. Pour the water into the inner corner of the eye nearest the nose so that it will flow across the eye and out its outer edge. In case only one eye is involved, this method will prevent the chemical from getting into the unaffected eye.

After the chemical has been thoroughly washed out of the eye, put several drops of clean vegetable or mineral oil into the eye. Do not try to use a neutralizing solution and chemical antidotes for acids or alkalis; more harm than good can result from their use. Cover the eye with a sterile gauze compress, bandage it in place, and get your injured child to a physician promptly.

Electric Burns

Burns of this nature may follow contact with an electric apparatus, a bolt of lightning, or with a charged electric wire which frequently is put in the mouth by infants and can result in severe burns and scarring of the lips and mouth. Electric burns are varied in type. From their appearance alone, it is impossible to tell how serious it is. Lightning burns show a feathering pattern and recognition of this type of burn can be important in a child that is in coma. Even delayed resuscitation can be successful.

Burns with a small surface sometimes char and destroy the tissue for an inch or two along the path of the current's discharge. *First aid treatment to the burned area is of small consequence, since the most serious phase of electric injury*

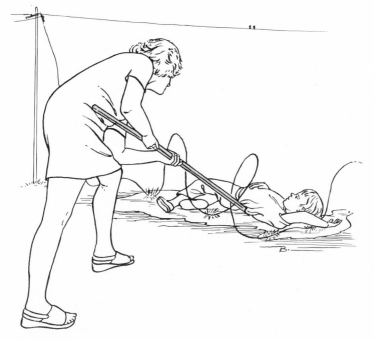

If your child is in contact with a live electric wire or other source of electric current, he must be separated from it.

is the damage inflicted on the heart and respiratory center, either of whose functions may be impaired.

The child must be freed from contact with the electricity as soon as possible. Use a dry stick, rope, coat, or other *dry* nonconductor of electricity. When possible, the electric current should be interrupted at once by pulling the main switch or the plug from the socket.

If respiration has ceased, artificial respiration should be started immediately and continued until medical help is obtained and the child's condition determined. Prevent contamination by covering the burned area with a sterile or clean cloth.

Most electrical burns, in children, occur in the home where current is supplied under low voltage and the severity of the burn happily is less than when high voltage is involved, as occurs in many industrial accidents.

Electric Shock

Rescue. If your child is still in contact with a live electric wire or other source of electric current, he must be separated from it. **Do not use your bare hands.** You might get a severe shock yourself. Shut off the current, preferably by pulling the main switch in your switchboard if it is quickly accessible. Otherwise, yank the cord from the socket. If you can't do either, then pull the live wire away from your child by using a dry stick, rubber gloves, dry cloth, rolled-up newspaper, or paperbag wrapped around your hand. If you have to pull the child himself away, don't touch him with your bare hands. Use folds of cloth or newspaper, rubber gloves, or a pole or board —anything that is not metal and is dry.

Treatment. Give your child artificial respiration immediately, call a doctor, and give first aid treatment to his burns as soon as possible (see pp. 169, 179).

DANGEROUS MEDICAL SITUATIONS 16

In this chapter we will discuss medical situations which usually are not life-threatening—that is, breathing and circulation have not been interrupted and bleeding is able to be controlled. These situations are:

1. Wounds
2. Bites
3. Fractures of the bones
4. Head injuries
5. Dislocations

6. *Miscellaneous*
   Leg cramps
   Embedded objects in eye, ear, nose, throat
   Tooth injury
   Sprains

The *general guidelines* for these situations are not the same as for those which are life-threatening. When you have perhaps only four minutes in which to save a child's life, you must react quickly using whatever knowledge you have: it is worth at least a try even though your actions may not be professional. With the situations we will discuss in this chapter, errors in technique and judgment should be avoided. Such mistakes can result in further injury. The purpose of care and treatment for these dangerous but not necessarily life-threatening situations is to maintain your child in the best condition possible until medical attention can be obtained. Unless your child must be moved out of immediate danger, it is best to give first aid on the spot. Let him be moved by persons trained to do so.

The injured child is generally frightened, sometimes incoherent, and in need of the gentle, steadying influence of an understanding and competent person. Putting the mind of an injured child at ease—reassuring and comforting a panicky child—is often a crucial part of treatment.

Check your child for signs of shock and treat as needed (see p. 172). It is usually a good idea to cover any injured child with a light blanket: shock may be delayed and show up later.

Carefully examine your child to identify hidden injuries in addition to the obvious ones. Once you think you know what injuries are present, call for help which would be appropriate for the injury. For example, children with wounds can generally be transported by the rescuer as long as bleeding control can be maintained while in transit. On the other hand, children with bone fractures of certain kinds, should be moved only by trained persons.

Wounds

All wounds are referred to as either open wounds or closed wounds. Be able to describe the wound when you call for professional help.

Open Wounds

Open wounds are wounds in which the skin has been cut or torn. These are divided into four major groups.

1. Abrasions (Scrapes). These wounds are caused when the skin is rubbed or scraped off and there are irregular, superficial injuries of the skin. Usually, little bleeding occurs unless the abrasion is very deep. An example of this type of wound is a skinned knee. (Be sure, however, that the wound is superficial and does not go to the bone. In this event, immediate medical help is needed.)

Abrasions often contain bits of grease, gravel, or other foreign matter, which are ground into the skin. If this debris is not removed, a serious infection could develop and a permanent tattoo-like scar might result. If the abrasion is not deep, the foreign matter can be flushed away with antiseptic solutions, such as fresh hydrogen peroxide or sterile (boiled and cooled) water, followed by gentle washing with soap and water. Careful cleansing of the wound is important, since abrasions are easily infected.

After cleaning, cover the wound with a single layer of non-adhering (will-not-stick) gauze or a sterile pad and fasten in place with adhesive tape. If the gauze tends to stick when you change the dressing, soak the gauze for a few minutes with fresh hydrogen peroxide solution or with a solution of one teaspoonful of salt to a quart of boiled and then cooled, or sterile water. Professional care is not usually required unless the area involved is very large or deep so that foreign matter cannot be removed by the techniques described. It is also important to watch the healing process and make sure infection does not develop.

2. Incisions (Cuts). These wounds are made by sharp, cutting objects such as knives, razor blades, or broken glass. Tetanus infection (or lockjaw) is a constant danger and tetanus booster injections are always to be considered.

Deeply incised wounds may bleed profusely because an artery or vein may have been cut. Nerves, muscles, and tendons may also be damaged. First, pressure must be applied to control bleeding and then the wound should be covered with a sterile dressing and bandaged. *If there is no evidence of bone fracture* and the bleeding open wound is on the hand, arm, leg, or foot, the injured extremity should be raised above the level of your child's heart. Medical aid should be sought immediately, especially if the wound is deep to the bone.

Less serious superficial cuts should be treated by non-sticking dressings taped in place. If the wound edges gape or are visibly open, they may be drawn together by using the butterfly strip technique (see p. 257). If healing does not progress rapidly or if there is any evidence of swelling, increased tenderness or redness, or streaks extending outward from the wound, it is probable that infection has occurred, and a physician should be consulted promptly.

3. Lacerations. Wounds of this type are made by striking with or falling against a blunt object, or by a ragged tearing of the tissues. Frequently lacerations are combined with contusions and are called *contused lacerated wounds*. Going through a windshield in an automobile accident usually produces this type of wound. Running with a glass in the hand and then tripping can produce a severe laceration and bleeding. Scalp laceration wounds, even minor ones, bleed profusely. Using any sterile or clean cloth with firm pressure for a few minutes will control most of these bleeding wounds. Stitches or trimming the hair about the site is usually unnecessary.

Like abrasions, lacerations may contain foreign matter which should be cleaned in order to prevent infection and to ensure proper healing. Soak the wound with fresh hydrogen peroxide or sterile water and then gently wash it with soap and water; make sure to wash dirt away from the wound and not into it. When lacerations are extensive (as from automobile accidents), do not attempt to treat them at the site of the accident. Simply cover the injured area with a thick sterile or clean dressing, tape firmly in place, and get your child to a hospital as quickly as possible.

If the laceration is not too large or deep, the edges may

be drawn together by means of a "butterfly strip" (see p. 257). This technique is both timesaving and painless and is especially useful for children who are apprehensive even though the type of wound does not require stitches.

Newly marketed skin closures with fabric backing and special adhesive can be used (ask your druggist) for closing of minor wounds, eliminating the need for suturing with needles.

4. Puncture Wounds. A puncture wound results from penetration of the skin and underlying tissues by a sharp object. For example, stepping on a nail will produce a puncture wound. Puncture injuries are also caused by needles, points of knives, bits of wire, and large splinters of wood, metal, or glass. Bullets make puncture wounds, as do bits of glass or other debris blown into the air by an explosion. Firecrackers can also cause puncture wounds. Flying debris from power mowers can puncture skin and deeper structures.

Examine the wound carefully. Note size of the surface area of the wound, and try to estimate its depth. Observe all possible details about the object which produced the wound so that you can report them to the attending physician. It is especially important to see if a part of the object has broken off and become embedded in the wound. *All puncture wounds should be seen by a physician.*

If the blood flow is limited, encourage bleeding by gentle pressure about the wound. Do not squeeze hard; avoid bruising the wound or the area around it. Do not probe into the injury. If a large object, such as a big splinter, is still in the wound, do not try to remove it; the attempt might cause severe bleeding.

Do not try to clean the wound. Apply a protective dressing to the injury and fix in place with adhesive tape. Treat for shock unless the wound is small and shock is unlikely.

Puncture wounds generally differ in two important

ways from other types of open wounds. First, bleeding from a puncture wound that is restricted to the outside of the skin is likely to be limited (unless the scalp is involved) since the opening at the surface is usually small. Internal bleeding and damage to important organs may occur in major puncture wounds. Second, the risk from infection is likely to be greater than in cuts or incised wounds. Germs are dragged deep into the wound by the penetration object, and because there is little, if any, free bleeding, germs are not readily "washed" out of the wound. Furthermore, the small surface opening tends to shut air out of the depth of the wound. *Always remember that tetanus (lockjaw) is a special hazard in any puncture wound.*

Repeat: all puncture wounds, even though minor, should be seen by a physician, and a booster tetanus toxoid or antitoxin injection given, if indicated. Tetanus is an extremely serious disease, easy to prevent but very difficult to treat.

Closed Wounds

Closed wounds are wounds in which there is no break in the skin. The tissues beneath the skin are damaged, sometimes severely, but comparatively little evidence of this damage shows on the surface, such as evident bleeding. Closed wounds may range from minor bruises, such as a black eye, which cause only temporary discomfort, to severe crushing injuries which can be a serious threat to life. Motor vehicle accidents and severe falls are examples of causes of such latter injuries.

Examine the wound carefully, without touching it. Try to determine the seriousness of the wound. A "black eye" can be treated simply by cold applications. Anything more serious must be seen by a physician.

Handle the injured child gently. Rough or unnecessary handling causes pain and increases danger from shock.

Do not move your child if he is already lying down —unless he must be taken away from danger such as fire or falling debris or unless he must be transported to medical aid. Look carefully for other injuries. Treat for shock.

Bites

Snake Bites

Snake bites cause acute anxiety and fear both for the bitten child and those who come to his help. *Snake bites are not common and, when they do occur, the victim has a very large chance of recovery*, if immediate treatment in given. This treatment has three objectives:

- Reduce circulation of blood in the bite area.
- Delay absorption of the snake venom.
- Maintain breathing and reduce anxiety.

If you are within 30 minutes' drive of medical assistance, *take your child at once to the medical facility.* During transport, keep the child quiet and *immobilize* (no movement) the bite area, keeping that area below the level of the victim's heart. *Cold cloths* placed over the wound will slow absorption of the venom. Watch for signs of shock. Keep your child warm; offer any *non-alcoholic* liquid if your child can swallow easily. Give artificial respiration if necessary.

Symptoms from the bite can include dizziness, vomiting, loss of vision, substantial swelling near the bite, excruciating pain, and unconsciousness.

If you are *not* within 30 minutes of medical assistance, you must take action to remove the venom:

- Wrap a wide tourniquet from two to four inches *above* the wound. This tourniquet should be firm enough to delay the spread of venom, but not tight enough to stop blood flow completely.

- If possible, have the bite area free of any movement and below the level of the heart (lowered but not elevated).
- Make incisions with a sterile blade at fang marks and over the probable venom deposit points. Incisions should be about ½ inch long an ⅛ inch deep and should follow the *long axis* of the arm or leg. DO NOT MAKE CROSS-CUT INCISIONS.
- Suction by mouth or syringe should be started promptly on these incisions and continued for 30 to 60 minutes. If you use your mouth, do not swallow the venom; rinse your mouth, if possible.

The bitten child should be kept quiet and warm to prevent shock and then taken to a hospital or physician immediately after first aid. If the snake can be safely killed and stored, it should be taken along so that medical personnel can have it identified to determine the specific antivenom needed. Pit vipers are responsible for the great majority of all snake bites in the United States and the antivenom is readily available in emergency room facilities.

Snake bite kits, small enough to fit in a coat pocket, are available in pharmacies and should be carried by persons who are frequently outdoors in snake-infested areas not near prompt medical assistance.

Animal Bites

Animal bites may cause rabies, tetanus, or other serious infection. Consult a doctor immediately. Wash the wound under running tap water to flush out the animal's saliva; then wash the wound for five minutes with plenty of soap and water. Rinse the wound thoroughly with clear running water, and cover it with a sterile dressing fastened in place.

Avoid moving the injured part unnecessarily during transport to a medical facility. The physician can treat the wound more effectively and decide what measures are necessary to guard against rabies and tetanus infection.

If the bite is from an unknown dog, cat, or other animal, whose rabies inoculation cannot be quickly determined, be able to describe the animal so that it can be caught and turned over to the police or health department official for examination. If the animal cannot be examined for rabies, consult your physician as to the nature and circumstances of the bite and the advisability of having your bitten child receive the series of anti-rabies vaccine injections and serum. These injections are absolutely necessary if the animal has rabies.

Although dog bites are most common, cat bites also are frequent and often more dangerous because the mouth of a cat may contain a wider variety of bacteria beyond rabies. Many wild animals also transmit rabies: foxes, bats, raccoons, and skunks are the most common. Rabies is rare in small, wild rodents such as squirrels, chipmunks, rats, and mice, and anti-rabies treatment is rarely necessary.

Human Bites

Human bites should be treated promptly because of the severity of the infection which so often develops in the wound. Human mouth bacteria are varied and multiple and capable of producing serious infection in a badly lacerated or punctured wound. Irrigate the wound with clear running water and then wash with soap and water. A sterile dressing should be applied. Seek medical attention as soon as possible for any human bite. Although human bites are not common, they can lead to serious infections.

Fractures of the Bones

Fractures commonly result from falls in the home, during sports and recreational games, and automobile accidents. Knowing what to do—and what not to do—before medical help arrives may prevent crippling, and it may even save your child's life.

Fractures are classified as closed (simple) or open (compound). A fracture is closed if there is no wound at or near the site of the break. It is open if a wound accompanies the fracture, so that there is an opening between the broken bone and the outside of the body. Such a wound can be made by the jagged, razor-sharp edges of the broken bones which may puncture the skin from the inside. The wound also may be produced by a forcefully moving object such as a bullet or a knife.

Open fractures are more serious than closed fractures. There is likely to be considerable bleeding, and greater risk exists that jagged bone edges may damage the nerves, muscles, and blood vessels around the fracture. There is also the added danger of infection, since germs can enter through the open wound. Shock is likely to be present and should be treated. (See pp. 172-173.)

General guidelines for dealing with fractures (or suspected fractures) include the following:

1. Call for medical help immediately, but do not delay in examining your child carefully and gently. The least carelessness, or rough or improper handling, can quickly change a closed fracture to an open one by dislodging the bone fragments and driving them through the tissues and skin at the site of the break.

2. Prevent any movement of the injured areas.

3. Control bleeding.

4. Provide immediate support in the form of a splint for the injured part.

5. *Do not move a person suspected of having a fracture*, and do not handle the injured part until the broken bone has been splinted.

6. *Do not attempt to set it.* The time-honored rule of "Splint 'em where they lie" must not be violated except in the direst emergency, when it may be necessary to move your child immediately away from fire, falling debris, or other hazards. Even then, do everything possible to keep the ends of the broken bone from moving.

Satisfactory splints can be made from anything that will keep the bones immobilized. Wood or metal materials are preferable, but in an emergency you can use umbrellas, tightly rolled magazines or newspapers, or even pillows or blankets.

When boards or other hard objects are used, they must be well-padded before they are placed against the injured part. Use cotton, clean rags, or other soft material for padding. Make splints long enough to reach beyond the joint above and the joint below the break in order to immobilize the broken bones. Secure splints with bandages or make improvised ties from handkerchiefs, belts, neckties, or straps. Fasten snugly but not so tightly that circulation is cut off. Leave fingers and toes exposed and extending beyond the end of the splint so that they can be observed for signs of swelling or color change. If these signs occur, loosen the splint slightly.

If the fracture is an open one, provide as sterile a protective dressing as possible for the wound to prevent germs and dirt from entering.

In fractures involving the fingers, hand, wrist, and forearm, it is important to remove rings, wrist watches, and bracelets promptly after the injury before swelling of the parts make their removal difficult.

Treat for shock. Shock of some degree usually follows every fracture, especially open fractures, and you should observe closely for any shock symptoms.

Fractured Neck

If you suspect a broken neck, your child must be transported on a rigid support, flat on his back **(face up)**. If he is not already lying on his back, he must be turned carefully to that position. This must be done as a coordinated effort by at least three persons so that his head and neck are kept at all times in line with the rest of his body, without any twisting. It is better to wait to turn the injured child on his back until the rigid support on which he will be transported is ready or available for use; then he can be turned and placed on the support in one operation.

An ordinary stretcher is not suitable for transporting a child with a broken neck, as even the firmest ones are too flexible. If you must move a child with a broken neck, the following procedures should be observed:

1. Procure a board or boards, at least 7 feet long and wide enough to amply accommodate the injured child. If

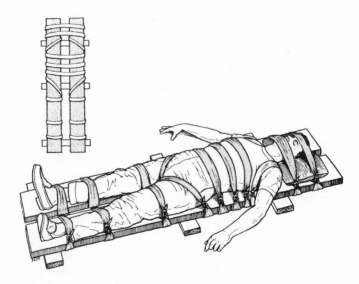

In an emergency, an improvised splint can be made to transport, in the face-up position, a person with a fractured neck.

two boards are used, leave a space of at least 2 inches between boards.

2. Unless the boards are heavy, they must be reinforced with cross pieces, nailed or tied crosswise at points corresponding approximately to where the person's shoulders, hips, and heels will be.

3. Pad the boards with blankets, and arrange ties in such a way that they may be tied over the victim at interval spaces so as to hold him absolutely firm and immobile during transportation.

4. Next, place the improvised stretcher as close as possible to the victim.

5. Assign one person to do nothing but hold the victim's head in order to keep it in line with the rest of the body at all times, or do this job yourself.

6. Assign one person to hold his shoulders; one, to his hips; and another, if available, to his legs and feet; if not, the one assigned to the hips will have to be responsible for the legs as well.

7. If there is insufficient help (at least four people) so that he can be lifted onto the stretcher, at a prearranged signal, gently lift the injured child just enough so that the stretcher can be slid under him.

8. Be sure that the entire body is moved as a unit, without any twisting of, or pushing or pulling on, the spine.

9. When the injured child is on the stretcher, secure him firmly with ties and cover him with blankets.

10. Do *not* use a pillow of any kind under the head, but *do* use sandbags, rolled-up newspapers, sweaters, or coats *on each side of the head* to keep it from moving during transit.

11. Someone should guard the injured child's head during the trip to the hospital to be sure that it does not move.

12. Neck injuries should never be minimized as only minor "whiplash."

Fractured Back

The procedures for caring for a child with a broken back are the same as those listed for one with a broken neck, *with this important exception*: the injured child must be transported in the **face-down position**.

The injury which produces a broken back often occurs when a child is bent forward so that he is often found lying on his abdomen. In that case:

1. Gently straighten your child's body with the same care and in the same way as for broken neck, but place him *face down* on a rigid stretcher.

2. If your child should be found lying wholly or partially on his back, apply the splint *before* turning him.

3. After the splint is firmly secured along *the front* of your child's body, he may then be safely and easily turned.

4. If it is not possible to do this, turn and place him on the stretcher as described for a broken neck, except that he must be placed in the face-down position.

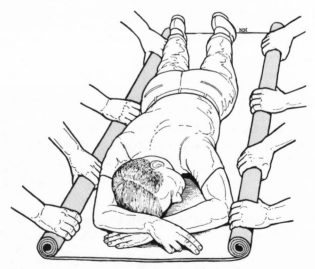

Using a blanket as a stretcher to carry a person with a broken back, with four persons carrying.

5. If nothing is available with which to make a rigid support, a blanket may be used to make a carry, but at least *four helpers* are needed if your child is to be lifted in this way.

6. If sufficient help or materials are not available to move an injured child, cover him with a blanket or coat and wait for adequate help.

It is better to do nothing than to do harm.

Head Injuries

Although your child may have been thoroughly examined following a fall (or trauma) for evidence of head injury, there are certain signs of trouble which may appear in the next 48 hours. Even though it has been considered safe to allow your child to return home from the hospital clinic, by the examining physician, observe your child carefully during the next 48 hours, and telephone your physician should any of the following signs of trouble develop.

Signs of Trouble:

1. *Excessive Drowsiness.* Your child may well be exhausted by the ordeal surrounding the injury, but he should be easily aroused by methods that you would ordinarily employ to waken him from a deep sleep. If you cannot do this, notify your doctor.

2. *Persistent Vomiting.* Children will, in most cases, vomit one or more times following a severe head injury. Should the vomiting recur more than once or twice, or should it begin again hours after it has ceased, notify your doctor.

3. If one pupil of the eye appears to be larger than the other, notify your doctor.

4. If the child does not use either arm or leg as well as previously, or is unsteady in walking, notify your doctor.

5. Should speech become slurred or the child is incoherent, notify your doctor.

6. If severe headache occurs, particularly if it increases in severity and is not relieved by aspirin, notify your doctor.

7. Should a child complain of "seeing double" or should you detect any failure of the eyes to move together appropriately, notify your doctor.

8. Should a convulsion occur place the child on his side in an area where he cannot fall, be sure there is ample room for his breathing, and place a firm object between the molar teeth to keep mouth open. Stay with the child. Have someone notify your doctor immediately.

On the night following the head injury, or during a nap, it is advisable to awaken your child (every two hours) and look for any of these danger signs.

Dislocations

Dislocations of joints and bones may be caused by a fall, by a blow against the joint, by a sudden twisting of the joint, or, less commonly, by a sudden contraction of the muscles which provide movement for the bones making up the joint. Most common dislocations are those of the shoulder and finger joints, with that of the elbow next in frequency. Bear in mind that a dislocation may be accompanied by a fracture of the bones near the joint. Handle all dislocations according to the general principles already discussed for closed fractures until the injury can be seen by a physician.

What To Look For and Do

- Swelling; discoloration; tenderness to touch

- Obvious deformity of the joint when compared with the uninjured counterpart
- Pain when movement is attempted or inability to move the joint
- Do not move the affected joint. Immobilize the area of dislocation as much as possible. Obtain medical attention.

Pulled Elbow (Nursemaid's Elbow)

This sudden and dramatic injury occurs in one-to-five-year-old children when one of their arms is extended and is then pulled sharply by an adult or an older child. It is caused by the sudden jerk of the arm when a child is picked up by the hand, pulled up the stairs or out of bed, swung around in a circle, or, when walking hand in hand, the child tries to run off and the adult holds firmly to his hand.

There is often a "popping" sound heard initially; then the child immediately starts to cry and refuses to use his arm, holding it limply at his side. He can move his fingers, but he cries harder if someone tries to manipulate the arm. He will not hold an object in the hand. The pain is not always in the elbow, however, and this makes it difficult to diagnose. The child may complain of pain in the shoulder, the collarbone, or the wrist, but, if pressure is put on the elbow, he winces in severe pain which thereby pinpoints the trouble.

The reason for this common occurrence is that the joints are very elastic at this younger age, and the head of the radius (the bone of the forearm that runs from the elbow to the thumb-side of the wrist) is small and still composed of cartilage instead of bone. About the age of five, the head of the radius changes to more of a club shape, grows larger, and becomes hardened to bone so it cannot easily slip out of place.

Putting the elbow back into its normal position (reduction of the pulled elbow) is relatively easy and requires no anesthesia. However, it should be done by a physician. Often this dislocation is "reduced" inadvertently by the parents with manipulation while putting on a sweater or coat, or simply by accidentally using the correct maneuvers while examining the involved arm. Usually there is an audible click, and pain ceases when this occurs and the child will again move his hand and arm normally.

Miscellaneous

Leg Cramps ("Charley Horse", "Growing Pains")

A "charley horse" is a sore muscle, usually in the legs, which has been exercised too strenuously or traumatized in some athletic event. Often, the calf of the leg is hard and may show a protrusion. The condition may persist for several days and treatment usually consists of rest, gentle massage above and below the affected area, and cold applications initially and then heat.

"Growing pains" in almost all cases are caused by fatigue in an overactive ("never still a moment") growing child. A small number of these children may be found to have poor foot mechanics (frequently, weak "flat" feet with knock-knees)—problems which often can be helped with corrective shoes.

Treatment for those who show no demonstrable cause for these pains is to make some attempt to curtail activities with rest periods and measures to relieve the pain, which usually occurs at late evening, often after the child is relaxed in bed. A hot bath at bedtime, with massage of the legs, will bring some relief. After a particularly active day, and for severe pain, a mild analgesic, such as aspirin, may be given. Persistent muscle and joint pains should be investigated by your physician.

Embedded Objects in Eye, Ear, Nose, Throat

Eye. The object may lodge on the inner surface of either the upper or lower eyelid or on the eyeball itself, or it may remain freely movable in the space between the eyeball and the eyelids. In any of these spots, it will painfully scratch the eyelid or the eyeball, or both, as the eye moves around. Such scratching will quickly set up an inflammatory reaction with reddening of the eyelids and eyeball, profuse tearing (crying), and an abnormal sensitivity of the eye to light.

First, wash your hands before touching the eye. Don't rub the eye. To do so may embed the foreign body in the eyeball. Bring the upper eyelid down over the lower one, and hold it there for a moment or two while your child is told to look upward. This will cause tears to flow which often will wash out the object. Release the upper lid.

If the foreign object has not been removed, carefully place the index and middle fingers just below the lower eyelid and gently pull the lower lid down. Look carefully at the inside of the lower lid for the object. If it is seen there, it can be lifted out carefully and gently with the corner of a clean handkerchief, facial tissue, or a small bit of sterile cotton wrapped around the end of a toothpick. Moisten the cotton slightly with water before touching it to the eyelid. CAUTION. *Do not try to remove a speck actually embedded in the eyeball, even if it is visible.*

If the object cannot be located on the inner surface of the lower lid, it may sometimes be flushed out by using an eyecup to wash the eye or a medicine dropper to flood the eye, with warm salt water (one-fourth teaspoonful of table salt to a glass of distilled water or boiled water cooled to body temperature).

If the above measures do not remove the object, put a few drops of castor oil, olive or vegetable oil, or medicinal mineral oil into the eye. If the foreign object is still present, consult a physician promptly.

Ear. Children, especially young ones, frequently poke beads, peas, paper, and other objects into their ears. Occasionally an insect may get trapped in the ear.

Do not try to remove anything that is not visible or smooth objects like beads. These are very likely to be pushed in even farther. It may be possible to grasp with tweezers a soft object (paper or cloth) which you can see. *Most objects lodged in the ear should be removed by a physician.*

Nose. Small children have been known to poke an incredible variety of small objects into their noses. Food, beans, peas, buttons, stones, clay are just a few examples. Also, children may occasionally be unwilling hosts to an insect which has inadvertently flown into the nose, where it may cause a burning, painful sensation.

Do not use water. Drop a little mineral oil or vegetable oil into the child's nose. This will quiet the frantic buzzing and movements of any insect and will help keep a pea, bean, or other seed from swelling. The oil will also soothe the irritated lining of the nose. Have your child blow his nose gently (not violently) after the oil has been inserted. Sometimes this will remove the foreign body. Do not attempt to remove a foreign body from the nose unless it is easily grasped. This is a job for a physician.

Throat and Mouth. Young children sometimes inhale food or swallow a variety of objects which lodge in the throat. When any of large material lodges in the lower air passages the victim will usually cough, a reflex protective mechanism. Sometimes the foreign material will be coughed up. If this does not happen quickly, use the Heimlich maneuver described on page 178. When bits of glass or small pins are swallowed, feed your child strands of cotton from absorbent cotton balls mixed with mashed potatoes, apple sauce, or other pureed food available. The object often will be safely eliminated.

Tooth Injury

In accidents involving the mouth, teeth should be checked by a dentist.

When teeth are whole, especially in a young child, they should be saved and brought with the child to the dentist, since it is now possible to reimplant them under favorable conditions. The extremely loose or completely unseated tooth in the unconscious child is better removed to prevent its inhalation into the lungs during transportation to a medical facility. If the child is conscious, the tooth should be left in place so that the nerve root is kept intact. Hemorrhage from a tooth socket can be controlled by local pressure of a small piece of cotton (saturated in hyrdogen peroxide, if available) over the socket or by the application of ice to the area.

Sprains

A sprain is an injury to the soft tissues that surround a joint, the point at which two or more bones come together. These tissues—*ligaments and tendons*—may be partially torn or stretched, but the bones remain in place. There may also be injuries to surrounding blood vessels.

The joints most frequently sprained are the ankle, knee, wrist, elbow, and spine, in that order. Sprains may vary in severity from an injury which causes only minor discomfort to one which requires weeks of care before the joint can again function normally.

It is often very difficult to tell the difference between a sprain and a fracture at or near a joint. In fact, both may result from the same injury, and only a physician can rule out the possibility of a fracture. If there is any suspicion that a facture may be present, use first aid measures described for fractures and call a physician. As a rule, adhesive tape should not be applied. Elevate the sprained member, apply cold compresses, and then heat when it is comfortable.

What To Look For

- Pain in the injured joint. This is increased if movement of the joint is attempted.
- Tenderness to the touch about the injured joint.
- Rapid swelling of the joint. This is likely to be quite extensive if the sprain is severe.
- Discoloration over and about the joint. Black and blue marks beneath the skin are sometimes quite noticeable in moderate or severe sprains. Discoloration may not develop for hours or days after the injury, but may remain for weeks before fading.

What To Do

1. Rest the injured joint. For example, if the ankle joint is sprained, have your child get off his feet so that the joint is not moved or required to bear any weight.

2. Elevate the injured part. For *ankle sprain*, have your child lie down, and then place pillows or folded-up clothing under the leg and ankle so that the ankle is about 12 inches higher than the rest of the body.

If an ankle sprain occurs when you are unable to carry him to medical aid, put on an ankle bandage. It will provide support for walking. (See bandaging, pp. 254-56). Do not, however, use the bandage or try to have him walk if there is any other way to reach help. A sprained ankle may be a fractured ankle as well, and putting weight on broken bones can be disastrous.

For *knee sprain*, place a pillow or other padding under the leg so that it is raised. For *wrist sprain*, put the arm in a sling. Adjust the sling so that the fingers are about four inches higher than the elbow. For *elbow sprain*, put the arm in a sling.

For *back sprain*, use great care in handling or moving the injured person. If a fracture accompanies the sprain, this is a very serious injury. Give first aid as directed for back fracture (see p. 198) until the injured person can be seen by a physician.

Apply an ice bag or cold compresses to the injured joint. Cold will help contract the many tiny blood vessels about the joint which are sometimes damaged at time of injury. Leakage of blood and fluid from them adds to the swelling which accompanies a sprain. By contracting the tiny vessels, cold minimizes leakage and helps lessen pain. Continue the cold applications, usually until the injured child can be seen by a physician.

Do not apply heat immediately after injury, since it will increase leakage from tiny blood vessels, and add to swelling and discomfort. Some hours or a day after the injury, when the damaged vessels are sealed off by blood clotting, it is safe to switch from cold to hot. The exact time depends in general on the extent of the injury (the more severe the sprain, the longer the application of cold compresses) and the comfort of your child. He may find that the continuation of cold applications causes discomfort, or that the application of heat too soon adds to his pain. *The general rule is to use cold applications early, hot ones later*—cold packs, however, can be used indefinitely if they are most comfortable.

If the injured joint does not return to normal within 48 hours and pain continues, have your child seen by a physician. This is necessary because there is always the possibility that a broken bone may accompany the sprain. Also, good medical care can lessen the period of disability from a sprain, and hasten the return of normal function.

Remember that a sprain may not be distinguishable from a fracture, except by X-ray.

SUDDEN SEVERE ILLNESS

17

Convulsions and Seizure Disorders

Convulsions are a symptom of some underlying trouble and not a disease. They may be caused by many unrelated conditions, particularly in young children. For example, a convulsion in a child may be indicative of an existing serious disorder or may herald the onset of an acute infectious disease. The convulsion may be of short or long duration or may recur in rapid succession; and a strong-willed child may bring on a convulsion by holding his breath deliberately until he turns blue in the face and lapses into unconsciousness. In so doing, he may set up a cycle which will perpetuate itself for some time. Any convulsion should be viewed as potentially serious until the discovery of the cause proves otherwise.

Often, you may be alone with your child when a convulsion occurs and cannot leave him immediately, even to summon medical aid; therefore, you should know how to handle the immediate situation until such time as further help can be sought.

Convulsions can be of all degrees of severity, lasting from a few seconds to many minutes. The convulsion takes the form of muscle spasms and twitching. It may involve the entire body (generalized) or only part of the body—face, arms, trunk, and legs (localized). The child is usually unconscious. If the convulsion is sudden, he may fall and injure himself. If the muscles of the face and jaw are involved, the mouth twitches and foams; if the tongue or cheek is bitten in the process, the foam becomes bloody. The breathing is loud and labored due to clenched jaws. Contraction of neck muscles interferes with the blood supply returning from the brain, and the face becomes congested and bluish in color. Convulsions are frightening and serious, but rarely fatal.

Epileptic Convulsions

When an epileptic convulsion occurs, it may come on suddenly but it is more often preceded by some warning. As the seizure begins, your child turns pale, his eyes may roll upward, he may utter a hoarse cry, and he may fall to the floor and lose consciousness. He may stop breathing momentarily, and his face will turn blue. He may bite his tongue because of convulsive movements of jaw muscles, and there may be an involuntary movement of the bowels and emptying of the bladder. As the convulsive seizure progresses, the muscular movements become jerky and the arms and legs may thrash about. At this stage, breathing begins again and the dusky color clears. There may be frothing about the mouth and the froth may be blood-tinged from the trauma to the tongue. The seizure usually subsides in a matter of minutes, and the epileptic child then may regain consciousness, become alert, or lapse into a period of quiet or restless sleep.

The chief aim of first aid is to prevent any injury during the convulsive movements. Nothing can be done to shorten the seizure, and nothing should be done to restrain convulsive movements. Ease your child to the ground if he did not fall at the start of the seizure. Leave him where he is unless he is in a place of danger (near moving machinery or fire, for example)—then move him gently to safety. Place a pillow or a rolled-up coat or other clothing under his head. Loosen the collar about his neck. Wrap a pencil, wooden clothespin, small stick, or spoon with a handkerchief or other cloth, and gently (*but not forcibly*) place it between the victim's teeth so as to prevent the biting of the tongue. Do not try to pry the mouth open or give anything by mouth during the convulsive seizure or after it, until full consciousness returns.

Watch your child if he lapses into a deep sleep or period of unconsciousness after the seizure, but do not disturb him. Unless your child is a known epileptic under medical supervision, call a physician at the beginning of the convulsive seizure. If the epileptic is under medical care, follow your physician's previous instructions. A typical epileptic seizure requires no particular care or hospitalization following recovery, except rest. The child should be spared embarrassment and his classmates made to understand the nature of his disease, so as to avoid ridicule and harassment.

While the cause for epilepsy is still unknown, most epileptics who carefully follow their physician's advice may remain relatively free from attacks through the use of the many varied anticonvulsive drugs which are now available. Epileptic children should be well instructed as to the nature of their condition so that they can cope with it realistically.

Non-epileptic Convulsions

Non-epileptic convulsion is like the epileptic seizure except for the degree and duration. It is usually much milder, and it terminates earlier. This type is seen most frequently in small children and is associated with acute infections of all kinds where there is a sudden marked elevation of temperature. Convulsions are seldom, if ever, caused by teething or overeating.

Treatment is similar to that given for epileptic seizures except that you should promptly try to reduce any high temperature. Wring out towels which have been soaked in cold water and apply them to the bare skin of your child; fresh, cool towels should be applied frequently until there is reduction of the fever. An ice bag or cold cloth to the head can be helpful. When cool water is not available, rubbing alcohol sponging can also be used, but do not prolong this method of cooling. Keep in mind the danger of alcohol intoxication in children by inhalation of the fumes.

After the convulsion has subsided, put your child to bed. Keep him as quiet as possible, since unnecessary movements or noise may bring on another seizure. Continue to use cold packs if the temperature persists until a physician is able to see your child to determine the cause of the convulsion and/or the temperature.

Breath Holding

Episodes of breath holding in children may sometimes lead to fainting or convulsive-like twitching. This results from temporary lack of oxygen to the brain. The frightened parents (even a physician not experienced in dealing with children) may think the child is having a sudden attack of epilepsy. Such, however, is improbable, and, except in very severe cases, the differentiation is easily made.

Breath-holding spells are often associated with temper tantrums and usually occur as the result of the child's frustration, parental friction, insecurity, fright, or punishment. Attacks of breath holding usually occur only in young children, most often between the ages of one and four years.

The usual sequence of events is that the child becomes mildly hysterical, hyperventilates by rapid breathing, and then stops breathing. If he holds his breath long enough, he will become somewhat cyanotic (turn blue). He may faint or spasmodically arch his back or twitch convulsively. Generally, these symptoms are not serious and of short duration. Any attempts to deal with your child during the attack will prove fruitless, *and threats of punishment only make matters worse.*

Generally, children tend to "outgrow" these attacks.

The *treatment* is simply to try to improve your child's emotional adjustment making every possible effort to understand your child's responses to his total environment. It is important to avoid those frustrations which produce anger and fright in your child which in essence is the underlying cause of breath-holding episodes. Basically, what the child is attempting to attain is security, emotional love, and recognition as an individual.

Other Sudden Illness

Children tend to develop acute illnesses abruptly. It is important to know some of the signs and symptoms which may help you distinguish between injuries and actue illness. If you are uncertain of the nature of the problem and it appears serious, call your physician at once.

Fever generally indicates some sort of infection. Very few accidents, including brain injuries, can produce fever in a short period of time.

Complete absence of breathing may mean that death has occurred, but, more often than not, the heart is still beating and life can be saved if resuscitation measures (see **pp. 169-171**) are begun immediately. *Irregular breathing* is encountered in many emergency traumatic and medical conditions such as an injury to the brain, a stroke, or poisoning. An *increase in the respiratory rate (fast breathing)* can be caused by obstruction of the respiratory passages, by heart diseases, drug poisoning, and occasionally simply by exhaustion or fright.

Unconsciousness or coma is a serious condition in which your child does not respond to any stimuli. This condition is found with head injuries, poisonings, epilepsy, and many other medical diseases.

Paralysis is most often due to medical conditions, although injuries to the brain and spinal cord should always be considered.

Vomiting may be due to infections, injuries, or poisonings. Vomiting of blood may indicate bleeding of an ulcer in the stomach or injury to the upper intestional tract. It is also seen with many types of poisoning, such as caustics, iron, fluorides, phosphorus, aspirin and many others. In an accident, there is always the possibility of blood from the injured mouth or nasal cavity being swallowed and later vomited.

Fainting. Individuals with minor injuries may faint simply from the sight of blood or a gaping wound. One who has fainted looks pale and is often covered with perspiration; the pulse will usually be slow. Recovery will occur promptly if the victim is allowed to lie flat with the feet elevated. Certain children and adults are predisposed to fainting easily, even under minor circumstances and stress.

Croup

Croup is a general term that applies to a variety of respiratory conditions in children usually occurring during the cold weather and winter months. Croup in itself is not a disease, but a group of symptoms, sometimes alarming, with the following general characteristics: a hacking cough which can be described as "barking"; hoarseness; and a croaking sound, called stridor, when the child takes in a breath. In spasmodic croup the typical cough and symptoms often begin in the late evening—sometimes called "midnight croup." Young children between the ages of one and three are frequently involved, although older children also can have croup. Some children have a tendency for croup and may continue to develop the symptoms for many years with each new respiratory infection.

Usually, but not always, the child at the outset has a mild cold with a runny nose and some cough. He does not particularly seem to be sick, fretful, or feverish, and eats normally. At bedtime everything seems to be in order. A few hours later, the child awakens with the characteristic "barking" and stridor sound: the voice is definitely hoarse and the child often is anxious and frightened.

At this point make a judgment. If the child can be calmed, so that he can breathe without undue strain, and if his skin and lips are reasonably pink, there is no immediate need for alarm. On the other hand, if the child's condition becomes worse after he has been awake for 15 minutes, if his lips and skin are dusky and bluish, and if he has trouble sucking in air, your physician should be called at once, regardless of the hour.

Most children without fever with acute spasmodic croup can be safely and effectively managed at home. Put the child in a closed bathroom, turn on the hot water shower or bath, and the steam often will improve and relieve the stridor and breathing distress. (Reading a story to the child while the steam is taking effect often helps calm him.) The same result has been noted by some parents as they take their child into the cold night air on the way to the physician's office or emergency room.

Inducing vomiting by tickling the back of the throat with a spoon or by giving an emetic (syrup of ipecac—½ to 1 teaspoon), may also relieve the stridor and spasmodic coughing.

Once some relief is obtained, the child should be returned to his bedroom, where a vaporizer—preferably cold air—should be in continual use. In the morning, there should be considerable improvement, although symptoms may return in a milder form again at night. It is wise to keep the child indoors and out of school until he has had at least one night free of symptoms.

Another and more serious type of croup is acute epiglottitis (the lid-like structure which automatically covers the opening to the larynx during the act of swallowing, to prevent food going into the larynx). While the common form of croup is viral, acute epiglottitis is due to a bacterial (most often *H. influenza*) infection. The onset is usually abrupt, being preceded by a minor cold, in about one-fourth of the sick. There is a sudden onset of moderate or high fever and difficulty in breathing. The older child will complain of sore throat and difficulty in swallowing. Severe breathing distress may begin within minutes or hours of the attack. Your child may stretch his neck to make breathing less difficult; an older child may prefer a sitting position, leaning forward with the mouth open and tongue somewhat protruding. Some children may progress rapidly to a shock-like state; showing pallor, cyanosis (turning blue), and impaired consciousness.

Acute epiglottitis is an emergency of the first magnitude, and it is imperative that your physician be called and medical attention be obtained immediately, preferably in an emergency setting where equipment and personnel for managing the respiratory obstruction is available.

Drug Abuse

There are at least five motives which may influence children to take drugs: (1) to prove courage by risk taking; (2) to act out rebellion and hostility toward society; (3) to facilitate sexual expression and performance; (4) to rise above loneliness and find emotional experience; and (5) to do what is the "in thing" of his friends.

Recognizing Drug Use. It is important that you recognize the common symptoms and signs of drug abuse, since many potential "hard core" young addicts can be rehabilitated if their involvement in drug abuse is detected in its early stages. Here are some useful clues for *recognizing drug use.*

Marihuana	Strong odor of burnt leaves on breath and clothes, dilation of pupils of the eyes, sleepiness, wandering mind, lack of coordination, craving for sweets, increased appetite
LSD HDMT DOM or STP PCP	Severe hallucinations, panic, feelings of detachment, incoherent speech, cold hands and feet, vomiting, laughing and crying jags, strong body odor, toxic psychosis and suicidal attempts
Amphetamines (pep or "up" pills)	Aggressive behavior, rapid speech, giggling and silliness, confused thinking, increased activity followed by fatigue, tremors, insomnia, no appetite
Heroin or morphine	Stupor, watery eyes, loss of appetite, needle marks on body, bloodstains on shirt, paraphernalia for injections
Glue sniffing	Drunk appearance, euphoric, incoordination, dreamy or blank expression
Barbiturates (down pills)	Stupor, dullness, blurred speech, drunk appearance, vomiting
Jimson weed (seeds) (atropine, scopolamine, hyoscyamine)	Hallucinogenic effect with agitation, confusion, disorientation, widely dilated pupils, elevated temperature, increased heart rate, dry mouth and flushed skin

Alcohol. More than 30% of the boys and 18% of the girls in American junior and senior high schools today are "heavy" drinkers—five to 12 drinks on at least one occasion per week—or "moderately heavy" drinkers, two to four drinks on at least one occasion per week according to a nationwide survey made by the Research Triangle Institute in North Carolina. This averaged out to nearly 25% of all students in grades 7 through 12. *Only 27% of all teenagers are teetotalers.* The preferred beverage was beer. The motives are similar to drug use.

The dangers of the accidental or intentional drinking of alcoholic beverages in children should never be overlooked or minimized. Many children have been made seriously ill, and a number of deaths have been reported from ingestion when children were unsupervised and had easy access to alcoholic products. Continuous alcohol sponging of a feverish infant has produced severe intoxication and even death from inhalation of alcohol vapors.

In acute alcohol poisoning, there is rather severe swelling and congestion of the brain and gastrointestinal tract.

Methyl, or "wood alcohol," causes blindness and other serious complications and many deaths. It is used as an antifreeze, solvent in shellac and varnish or paint removers.

Rubbing (or isopropyl) alcohol is an alcohol with added ingredients. It is an important industrial solvent and is also used as an ingredient of various cosmetics and for medicinal preparations for external use.

What To Do. If your child has had a significant amount of any alcohol, the physician should be called and notified of the type of alcohol taken, the amount if known, and the signs and symptoms, if any, that have developed. Do not assume that signs of intoxication ("drunkeness") will "wear off." Many alcohols are serious poisons in themselves, and often unsuspected drugs are taken as well. It is important, therefore, that treatment be started early to prevent serious or perhaps fatal complications.

Suicide. Suicide among young people has become a major health problem today. But because the subject has long been soft-pedalled in our society, few people know of the shocking increases in young suicides. Fewer still realize that many suicides can be prevented by the intervention and concern of others.

The school is involved in the problem of adolescent suicide and suicide attempts because it may be the site of the act or, more commonly, the place in which the child tells of his attempt or presents evidence of it, such as wrist lacerations. Among adolescent suicide attempts or gestures, the most common form occurring in the school is impulsive ingestion of medication which is available to the child. There may be witnesses to the act or he may tell friends or school personnel what he has done. Analgesics, sedatives, and tranquilizers are commonly used drugs.

A complexity of factors is responsible for the increase in young suicides. There are warning signs by which parents can spot suicidal feelings in a child. Generally, parents should be alert to a cluster of symptoms rather than any single factor. Here are some:

- Extreme withdrawal and isolation from others
- Deep and massive depression accompanied by an attitude of overwhelming hopelessness and helplessness
- Low self-esteem and feelings of worthlessness
- Threats of suicide and continual talk about death or wanting to die (more often in girls than boys)
- Suicidal gestures or attempts, no matter how minor
- Sudden change in personality and activities—failing in schoolwork, running away, becoming violently angry and disruptive
- Sudden heavy drinking or drug-taking

What To Do. Most important, take all suicide threats, gestures, or attempts seriously. Children who attempt suicide may just want attention; but without that attention they may well go on to more serious action.

Try to communicate with the suicidal child. Children may resort to suicide because they feel all other means of communication have been closed. Gather as much information as possible about the child's activities, thoughts or changes in attitudes and behavior from friends, teachers, classmates or acquaintances. Consult your physician for guidance.

The belief that talking about suicide encourages the act is a myth. People who are suicidal do not need to have ideas put into their heads. The ideas already exist. Learning where and how to find help may save their lives. And friends and family members can be the greatest help if they come to understand, rather than fear, the subject.

COPING WITH MINOR MEDICAL SITUATIONS

18

In this chapter we will mention several situations which frequently involve children and the medical seriousness of which is generally minimal. Most adults usually can provide whatever care is necessary. Follow-up professional care is often not necessary unless healing is not satisfactory, other symptoms develop, or if the adult caring for the child is not secure or satisfied with the care he is able to provide.

Bruises (Contusions)

Bruises are the most common of all injuries. Most of them are so minor that they pass unnoticed except for a little pain at the time of the injury. Others, however, such as the familiar black eye, can sometimes cause considerable pain and discomfort and should receive prompt first aid. If they are severe, they require medical attention.

A bruise occurs when a blow or a fall breaks some of the small blood vessels beneath the skin. Bruises may at first be reddish, but the color soon changes to a dark blue or purple. Later the discoloration changes to a brownish hue, then a yellowish one, and gradually fades out as healing takes place.

The blood clot which forms at the site of a contusion is called a *hematoma*. The typical signs are a raising of the skin (due to pressure of the accumulation of blood underneath) and softness to the touch.

Multiple bruise-like discolorations appearing without

any known injury require medical investigation.

In minor bruises, no treatment is necessary. In more severe bruises, first aid measures are aimed at limiting the swelling and discoloration and a lessening of the pain. Apply cold to the injured area immediately with an ice bag or cold compresses. Later, heat may be applied if more comfortable. Bruises of an arm or leg will be less painful if the limb is raised somewhat. If the bruise is accompanied by a break in the skin, proceed as directed in Wounds (see pp. 186-91).

In the case of severe bruise, the possibility of fracture or other damage to the underlying structures should be kept in mind. If the injury seems to be serious, your child should be seen promptly by a physician.

Dry-cold Applications

The most satisfactory device for applying dry cold is an ice bag. This can be improvised from a sturdy plastic bag such as that used for storing food in home freezers. The reusable chemical-ice packs which can be frozen in the refrigerator also can be used. Fill the bag with ice (never dry ice) a little more than half full. Wrap it in a hand towel or cloth and apply it to the affected area. Replace the ice as soon as it melts. Continue the treatment as directed by the physician or until the victim feels comfortable.

Moist-cold Applications

Moist cold is applied by means of compresses made from several thicknesses of gauze or clean soft cloth. They should be large enough to cover the affected area, and at least two are needed. Put a cake of ice or some cracked ice and water in a basin. (Do not use dry ice.) Lay the compresses on the ice or in the icy water. Protect any clothing or bedding with rubber sheeting or towels.

Wring out a compress or take it from the ice cake and place it on the affected area. Remove the compress as soon as it begins to get warm (usually in about three minutes), and replace it with another which has been cooling. Caution must be exercised in cases where the affected areas include some disturbance of circulation. If a physician has been consulted, follow his orders exactly in regard to the length of each treatment and the frequency with which applications are repeated.

Bruised Fingertip

One of the most common and most painful examples of a bruise results from hitting the fingertip with a hammer, slamming it in a door, or by the fall of a heavy object. Here, the bruise occurs under the fingernail, since the nail bed contains many tiny blood vessels that break easily. A small pool of blood, which accumulates under the nail, turns black within a few days, and the finger becomes extremely painful. The nail may loosen in time and come off as a result of the pressure and the direct injury caused by the blow to the growing part of the nail. There is a chance to save the nail, however, by promptly draining the accumulated blood from beneath it, but this requires treatment by a physician. So that the new nail will look better and the nail be less painful, do not attempt to pull off the nail if it starts to shed; fasten it in place with a small adhesive bandage until the new nail pushes off the old one.

Splinters

Children acquire splinters frequently. You should learn how to remove them. The following procedure is recommended: Wash your hands and your child's skin around the splinter with soap and water. Sterilize a needle and tweezers by boiling them 5 minutes in water, or in an emergency heating them in the flame of a match or cigarette lighter and then wiping off the carbon with sterile gauze or alcohol, if available. Loosen the skin around the splinter with the needle, and remove the splinter with the tweezers. Encourage slight bleeding by squeezing the wound gently. Apply a mild antiseptic solution, such as rubbing alcohol, and cover the wound with a sterile bandage.

Consult your physician if the splinter breaks or is deeply lodged. There may be need of a tetanus (lockjaw) booster injection.

Fishhook Accidents

What to do depends upon the size of the hook, its location, and the penetration. If the hook is small or medium-sized, if it has little penetration (just *up to* the barb), and if it is not in a critical spot such as the eye or

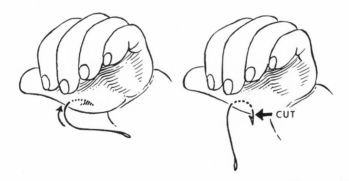

Fishhooks lodged in the hand can be best removed by backing the hook out of the skin. First, push the hook through the skin until you can see the barb. Cut the barb off and carefully remove the hook.

face, it is probably best removed by *backing it out of the skin*. If the hook has gone deeper and if the barb is embedded, it is best removed by a physician. But fishhook accidents usually occur in remote areas where first aid care is often all that will be available for some time. The hook should then be removed by pushing it through the skin until you can see the barb. Cut either the shank or the barb of the hook and remove the remaining portion from the skin. Clean and cover the wound. Because of the possibility of infection, including tetanus, a physician should be consulted as soon as possible.

Blisters

In general, leave blisters alone if they can be adequately protected against breaking. The fluid will be gradually absorbed by the deep layers of the skin, and the skin will soon return to normal except for possibly a little thickening at the site of the blister. However, if the blister is unusually large and is where it is likely to be broken by ordinary activity, it is best to have it opened by a physician.

If a physician is not available and if the blister should be drained, it may be opened in the following way: Gently clean the blister and the area immediately around it with soap and water by using gauze or cotton and being careful not to break the blister. Rinse well, and wash off the area with rubbing alcohol. Then puncture the edge of the blister with a needle that has been sterilized by holding its point in an open flame and wiped cleanly. Press the edges of the blister slowly and gently opposite the point of the puncture to force out the fluid. Cover it with a sterile gauze pad held in place with adhesive tape or a bandage.

If the blister has already broken, carefully wash off the

area with soap and water and apply a sterile gauze pad. Fix the pad in place with adhesive tape or a bandage. *Caution:* These first aid measures must not be used for blisters caused by burns. Such blisters should be left undisturbed as described in Burns (see p. 181).

Nosebleeds

Bleeding from the nose may be the direct result of a blow or the poking of fingers into the nose, or it may be caused indirectly by a number of other conditions such as high blood pressure (which is rare in children). Bleeding usually comes from only one side of the nose, and it most often comes from one of the small blood vessels near the surface of the partition (septum) which divides the nose. Frequent nosebleeds should always be called to a physician's attention.

Most nosebleeds will stop spontaneously. If bleeding continues, try the following first aid measures.

Have the victim sit up, hold his head back slightly, and breathe through his mouth. If he lies down, blood may run down the back of his throat where it cannot be seen, and bleeding may be considered stopped when it is not. Such swallowed blood may later be vomited and it should not be confused with bleeding from the mouth, stomach, or digestive tract.

Gently grasp the lower end of the nose between the thumb and index finger, and then firmly press the sides of the nose against the septum for about four or five minutes. Release pressure gradually. An ordinary spring-type clothespin may also be used in place of your fingers.

If pressure on the nose does not stop the bleeding, gently plug the bleeding nostril with a small strip of sterile gauze rolled up loosely (do not use cotton). Immersing the gauze in a common nose drop solution, if available, will increase the effectiveness of this procedure. Guide the strip of gauze slowly and carefully into the nose in a backward rather than upward direction. Leave about an inch of gauze sticking out of the nose so that it can be easily removed. Do not be in a hurry to remove the gauze when bleeding stops.

After bleeding has stopped, instruct your child not to blow his nose for several hours. Blowing could dislodge the blood clot that has formed and cause fresh bleeding.

If the nosebleed is not controlled by the above measures, consult a physician promptly.

Insect Stings and Bites

Children with a history of allergic reactions to insect stings should be under the care of a physician. You should always have on hand medication to be used to counteract the allergic reaction unless the child has been desensitized. Insect sting kits are inexpensive and readily available on the market. A highly allergic child can die in 5 to 30 minutes from a sudden allergic reaction to the sting of a bee, wasp, or hornet.

Even for a child with no history of allergic reaction who develops symptoms including shortness of breath, stomach pain, fainting and shock, medical treatment is needed quickly for this can be a serious emergency.

If the child has no history of allergic reactions to insect stings and shows signs of only localized discomfort in the area of the sting or bite, treatment should be provided to reduce discomfort. Wash the affected parts with soap and water. Apply a paste made of baking soda and a little water or use calamine lotion. Cover the bite with a cloth saturated with ice water if there is much swelling. A paste of meat tenderizer applied to the bite will often reduce the swelling and itching by its enzymatic action.

Ticks

Ticks are small, insect-like creatures about a quarter of an inch in length. They live chiefly in uncleared land, where they cling to grass stems, leaves, or branches until an animal or person comes along to which they can attach themselves. Dogs are symptomless carriers of infected as well as non-infected ticks. Once attached, ticks make a tiny wound in the skin with a sharp, rasplike "tongue," and they feed by sucking blood from their unwilling host. While they feed, they may also pass along germs of numerous diseases. Two of the most important of these are Rocky Mountain spotted fever and tularemia (rabbit fever).

Fortunately, only a small proportion of the tick population is infected with diseases that can be transmitted to man. There is no practical way, however, of telling which tick is infected and which isn't, so it is wise to avoid areas where ticks abound. If you live or vacation in these areas, take all possible precautions to avoid being bitten. A vaccine is available for Rocky Mountain spotted fever, and it should be administered to those living or working in infested areas, although it is not always effective.

Check the entire body for the presence of ticks whenever you have been exposed. Look carefully, especially behind ear lobes, about the head, neck, arms, and other hairy areas. Ticks can move so rapidly and lightly that they are usually not felt. It is important to remove ticks promptly, because the germs of some diseases (Rocky Mountain spotted fever, for example) may not be transmitted for as long as four to six hours after the ticks have attached themselves to the body and begun to suck.

Remove ticks by covering the insect with any available oil—salad, machine, mineral or vaseline. This prevents the tick from breathing. Usually the tick will disengage itself from the flesh quickly. If the tick does not disengage immediately, let the oil remain on the insect for about 30 minutes, then carefully remove the tick with tweezers. *Never remove or crush dog ticks by the fingers.*

Make sure all parts of the tick have been removed. Thoroughly scrub the bite area with soap and water. Dispose of the tick, preferably by burning or flushing down the toilet. Wash your hands thoroughly and sterilize the tweezers in boiling water.

If the victim becomes ill with fever, headache, and rash—which may erupt later—be sure to inform your physician of any tick bite he may have had. This will help the physician in his diagnosis, so that he can start the specific correct treatment early, preferably before the rash appears.

The best protection from ticks is wearing adequate clothing and inspecting the body thoroughly once or twice daily when in tick-infested areas. When venturing into tick-infested areas, wear high shoes, boots or leggings, and tuck trousers tightly into boots. Repellents sprayed on clothing can be quite effective in warding off ticks. Inspect the naked body carefully upon returning from a field trip, and remove the ticks.

In heavily infested tick areas, children should be inspected twice daily. Hang up field clothing in the open after returning home. Ticks still on your clothes will fall off eventually. Pet animals should wear flea and tick collars the year round.

Lice

Human lice occasionally enter a household by way of heads and clothing of children who have been infested at school or at the movies, on buses, and many other situations. Lice can be eliminated by heat treatment of clothing to kill the nits (eggs) and lice, and by scrubbing the hair and scalp with a 1% gamma benzene hexachloride (Kwell) preparation, which your physician often will prescribe on the phone.

Frostbite

When a part of the body, such as the fingers, toes, nose, cheeks, or ears, become frozen, the injury is called *frostbite*. It is caused by prolonged exposure to severe cold without adequate protection.

Do not let your child be exposed for long periods of time to severe cold. Cover his feet and hands, ears, and other exposed parts of the body with suitable clothing such as mittens, warm stockings, and earmuffs. Be extra careful when cold winds are blowing, since wind increases the body's rate of heat loss. Do not let your child get overtired in extreme cold; fatigue seems to predispose one to frostbite. Use particular caution about exposure to cold if your child has any condition which causes poor circulation of blood to his fingers and toes.

Try to warm up any part of the body that shows signs of numbness. Have your child wiggle his fingers or toes to increase the blood supply and thus warm them. Increase the amount of protective clothing which is covering the numb area. Place the cold part against another part of the body—for example, hand next to the chest.

Cover your child's frostbitten part with a wool scarf or other clothing, and get him indoors as soon as possible. Keep him warm. Give him hot tea.

If you are camping and cannot get indoors, place your body inside a sleeping bag or blankets, next to your child. It may be the only warmth available.

Do not rub the affected part. Do not put snow on it. Frozen tissues are quite fragile, and rubbing them may cause serious damage. The experience of arctic explorers and the results of military studies conducted in cold-weather conditions have shown that rubbing and applying snow increase the risk of tissue injury and gangrene. Handle with great care and gentleness.

Warm any frozen part by immersing it briefly in lukewarm (not hot) water (about 108°F is the correct temperature). Do not use hot water, hot-water bottles, or heat lamps because they will increase tissue damage. Keep the affected part away from intense sources of heat such as stoves, fireplaces, radiators.

Once affected fingers and toes are rewarmed, encourage the frostbitten child to exercise them. Do not disturb blisters if they develop. Consult a physician if necessary.

Sunburn

Always be careful about sun exposure, especially for an infant. To begin sunning, allow the baby about two minutes of sun each day, front and back; gradually increase this time, until after a month about 45 minutes of moderate sun exposure is allowed. Do not expose the infant to midday sun (best time is before 10:00 a.m. and after 3:00 p.m.). If the baby does get a mild sunburn, apply his skin cream or lotion, vaseline or petroleum jelly; see that clothing is light and airy; and keep him out of the sun. If the sunburn is severe, contact your physician.

Most commercial sunscreen preparations are formulated to permit tanning while avoiding burning. No sunscreen preparation will prevent sunburning if you stay out in the sun too long or if the preparation is removed by profuse sweating or various activities such as swimming. Sunning always should be moderate and gradual. Long exposures to the sun can cause severe medical problems.

Burns from sun lamps can be serious. Always read and follow carefully the instructions given by the manufacturer.

Heat Exhaustion and Heat Cramps

Children will sometimes develop symptoms of heat exhaustion and heat cramps after long periods of vigorous activity when temperatures are high. Heat exhaustion and cramps may occur together or separately. Your child should be taken to a cooler location and placed in a resting position. Gently massage cramped muscles, offer a few sips of salt water (one-fourth teaspoon of salt per glass) every few minutes for about an hour. If your child vomits do not offer salt water. In severe and unresponsive cases it may be necessary to seek medical assistance, primarily to assure proper replacement of lost body fluids.

Teach your child to avoid extended strenuous activity or exercise in temperatures nearing 100° Fahrenheit.

Hives

The simplest way to prevent hives is to avoid any food, drug, or plant which has previously caused a reaction. If you know your child is sensitive to a serum, vaccine, or a drug, you should volunteer this information to any physician who is caring for him.

Smooth, slightly elevated, pinkish or reddish patches (wheals) suddenly develop on the skin. These vary greatly in size—they may be just a dot or larger than a dime. They usually have a white center and are often irregular in shape. An intense stinging, burning, or itching sensation occurs at the site of each hive.

Bathe the wheals with a soda solution using three teaspoonfuls of baking soda to one glass of cold water. Apply the solution with a small pad of gauze or other cloth. Calamine lotion (obtainable at a pharmacy) will also often help relieve the itching and burning. Consult a physician if the hives are not relieved by the above treatment. If difficulty in breathing or swallowing should develop, call a physician immediately.

Hiccups

Hiccups, for a short while, in infants after feeding are normal and require no treatment. There is no sure way of preventing hiccups. In children, they may be brought on by a variety of conditions: indigestion, eating too rapidly, eating too much, and drinking carbonated and alcoholic beverages. Hiccups may also accompany, or be a complication of, a number of diseases.

Try these first aid measures in succession. Have your child hold his breath as long as possible; this often stops mild attacks. If this is not successful, have him grasp the end of his tongue with the fingers and gently pull it out of his mouth as far as it will go without producing discomfort. Usually he can do this for about 1-2 minutes.

If hiccups persist, have the victim drink a glass of plain cold water or a glass of cold water to which ½ teaspoon of baking soda has been added. If the hiccups still persist, have the child hold a *paper bag* tightly over his nose and mouth, and breath in and out of it for one to two minutes. Do not try scare tactics. On the other hand, be comforting and assuring.

If none of these measures is successful within a reasonable period of time, consult a physician.

Toothache

Beneath a tooth's tough, hard outer covering—the enamel—is a softer substance called the pulp. Embedded in this pulp are sensitive nerves which react quickly with pain when stimulated with heat, cold, pressure, or other irritation. Pain also develops if the nerves are irritated as a result of tooth decay.

If toothache occurs in the day time and a dentist is available, go for treatment at once. If toothache occurs at night, or if a dentist is not available, take these first aid measures: Look into the mouth under a good light. If there is a cavity in the aching tooth, clean it out by picking at it gently with a toothpick wrapped at the point with a wisp of sterile cotton. Saturate a tiny bit of sterile cotton with oil of cloves (obtainable at a pharmacy) and pack it gently into the cavity with a toothpick. Take care not to spill the oil of cloves on the tongue or inside the mouth; it will cause a burning sensation. Aspirin may be given for the pain.

If no cavity is visible in the tooth, or if the packing does not relieve pain, put an ice bag against the jaw on the side of the affected tooth. Sometimes a hot water bottle will be more effective; try one and then the other. Consult a dentist just as soon as possible, even if pain has been temporarily relieved.

Sleepwalking

The phenomenon of sleepwalking is poorly understood and the cause of sleepwalking is unknown. It is seen mainly in children, with boys outnumbering girls and is not a serious phenomenon; usually it disappears as the child grows older.

Sleepwalking is not to be disregarded, however, as tripping and falling can cause injury. A sleepwalker should be led gently back to bed. Upon awakening, sleepwalkers rarely have any recollection of what they have been doing.

Stomachache

Almost all children experience stomach pain at some time, and many have repeated stomachaches that are of grave concern to parents. No one recurring symptom presents so much uncertainty and concern for the physician. Stomach pain that is short-lived and not accompanied by other symptoms, and where the physician's examination and laboratory tests are within normal limits, are episodes usually of no serious consequence.

Vomiting and/or diarrhea, which are so common and often seasonal in most communities, are usually easily diagnosed ("it's going around") and managed. Yet this is not the time for parents to be complacent or to procrastinate. Any acute or prolonged bout of vomiting and diarrhea, with or without stomachaches, should be reported to your physician.

Acute appendicitis, in young children, is often a treacherous condition, and can occur during epidemics of "intestinal flu" as well as in normal times. It too, usually begins with some nausea, vomiting and sometimes diarrhea, but again all of these symptoms may be absent or obscure. There is always pain and tenderness in the abdomen, but sometimes the pain is so minimal that it does not manifest itself as a major symptom and can be easily overlooked. Although typically the pain of appendicitis is in the right lower part of the abdomen, it can also involve other parts of the abdomen and be confusing.

Appendicitis is usually seen in older children from 6-14 years, in more boys than girls. Fortunately it is relatively infrequent in infants and young children, where the diagnosis is often difficult because the child is unable to localize the pain with any accuracy. Any great delay in diagnosis and removal of the acute inflamed appendix can readily produce rupture, particularly in the thin-walled appendix of the young child, and subsequent serious peritonitis.

Recurrent stomachaches without detectable disease of the urinary or gastrointestinal tract, however, are a frequent complaint of children, particularly in the age group of 6 and 10 years. These attacks may go on for years, and are often emotionally upsetting to the child, discouraging to his parents, and diagnostically and therapeutically frustrating to the physician. Much patience and understanding are required.

When your physician has assured you that physically nothing is wrong, emotional tension and stresses may account for the pain. Treatment consists of reassurance and helping the child gain insight into the nature of whatever problem may be bothering him. Implying bluntly that the stomachache is "unreal", "made up", or "in the head" must be carefully avoided by parents and physicians alike: the pain is real. Glib statements that the stomachaches are psychological or emotional in character are difficult for parents to accept, unless the causes can be well described and attacked.

It may be helpful to compare this type of stomachache to headaches. Most everyone has headaches of one kind or another, and they know for sure that the headache pain is not imaginary even if there is no underlying sinus trouble, brain tumor, or high blood pressure. The pain of a stomachache, like headache, is always real but usually not serious.

A FINAL WORD

Most children are born naturally equipped to learn about the world around them. They have 330 paired voluntary muscles, 5 senses and one insatiable curiosity. When they reach the toddler stage this equipment begins to operate in an organized and intense way. By *child-proofing* the home only, no matter how completely, you are taking an unrealistic and negative approach to the toddler stage of childhood.

Homes need to be *child-oriented*. The basic idea of child-orienting is simply this: if a child has reached the decision, either verbally or through action, that he wants to do it himself, look for ways to make that decision a reality. For example, if your child is always emptying kitchen cabinets, he has obviously mastered the art of opening the cupboards. Instead of begrudgingly clearing away the mess and locking all the cupboards in retaliation, arrange a cabinet which contains unopened boxes and cans, pots, and safe utensils. By changing the contents of this special place, you can maintain your child's interest and, at the same time, reduce the chances that he will explore areas that are off-limits.

Child-orienting is an attitude, a perpetual use of the environment, not a single adjustment in your home for a short period, and it needs a commitment from you. It asks you continually to evaluate your home environment from the point of view of the child. What can he touch? What can she see? With a change here and there, what can they explore and do safely? Stay in tune with your infant's world; get down on your hands and knees and crawl where he does. You may be amazed at the "deadly treasures" you can find. What has rolled under the dresser? Have you looked under your couch recently? Besides dust, you may find pins, paper clips, bits of stale food, or even exposed springs that are just in the right location to injure the crawler's eyes.

The parent is the child's first teacher. You child's learning process and educational experiences can be best developed and expanded in a *child-oriented* home. In such an environment, there is a greater opportunity for optimal child growth and development with mastering of good health and safety habits, so that your child may reach the full potential of life in spite of the countless obstacles that will surround him. In this regard, we have tried, in this book, to emphasize the positive approaches and attitudes which parents must develop and share with their children:

- **PROTECTION**
- **DISCIPLINE**
- **REGULATION**
- **TEACHING**

PART FIVE

Ready Reference Guide

CONTENTS

How To Make an Emergency Phone Call

√ List emergency phone numbers (see First Aid Chart).

√ If these numbers are not immediately available when an emergency occurs, don't waste time.

√ Dial the Operator and say "This is an emergency." Ask for an ambulance and be prepared to give the following information.

- Your name and the phone number from where you are calling.

- *Your exact location:* Street name and house and/or apartment number and floor. If your location may be difficult for the ambulance to find, describe some nearby landmark or well-known street intersection nearest your location. Also, be sure your house number is visible from the street. At night, turn outside lights on, if available.

- Identify the emergency: for example, fire, convulsion, poisoning, severe bleeding, heart pains, fall, unconsciousness.

√ Learn to dial the operator even when there are no lights. Feel for the hole just underneath the finger-stop on a dial phone. On a pushbutton phone, feel for the middle button in the bottom row. Practice doing this with your eyes closed.

√ Teach your children and babysitters the proper way to call for help.

How To Get a Doctor

√ *At Home.* Keep your regular physician's telephone number posted beside your phone. Ask him to recommend two substitute doctors who may be called when he is not available. List their numbers too. If you can't get a doctor, call the police or other local emergency facilities.

√ *On the Road.* Telephone the police or hospital in the nearest town. For speed, dial, "O." Tell the operator, "This is an emergency call," and ask her to place the call. If there is no telephone nearby, hail a passing motorist and ask him to make the call as quickly as possible. When calling, always state your location on the road—route number, estimated distance from town, nearest landmark.

√ *In a Strange City.* Ask the hotel or motel management to call a doctor or hospital, or ask the telephone operator to call a doctor. In most cities, telephone companies maintain an emergency service in cooperation with the local medical society.

√ *Traveling Abroad.* If there is time, call the U.S. Embassy or the U.S. consulate and ask for the name and telephone number of a recommended doctor. Before you go abroad, you may wish to become a member of the International Association for Medical Assistance to Travelers, 745 Fifth Avenue, New York, New York 10022. All members receive a free directory which lists more than 200 participating hospitals and telephone numbers where a person can reach an English-speaking physician who is on call 24 hours a day. If anyone in the party is on regular daily medications, be sure to take an ample supply to last until the return home. Always include a basic first aid package.

How and When To Phone Your Physician

Ask your physician beforehand when is the best time for you to make non-emergency calls. If possible, save all your questions for then. Perhaps he has a set phone hour open for any and all calls. Don't call your physician outside of office hours unless your child's problem is urgent and cannot wait. A listing of situations in which you must call immediately is given on the following pages. When you call during office hours, your physician can advise you more fully because he has all the information on your child's record in his office. Here is a checklist of things you should do before you call.

√ If your child is sick, always try to take his temperature and pulse rate before calling for advice (see pp. 256-263).

√ Have first-hand knowledge of the child's condition.

√ Have a pencil and paper ready when you phone to write out instructions your physician gives you.

√ Make a list of the questions you want answered before you call.

√ Have the telephone number of the pharmacy on hand so your physician can order a prescription if necessary.

√ Be prepared to tell the person who answers the phone exactly what is wrong. Unless it is a medical emergency, you can often get advice you need without talking to your physician personally. Your message will get through and the physician will send one back, or call back when he can.

√ Be specific, if possible. Use words which have clearly understood meanings. Instead of saying "He has a fever", say, "He has a temperature of 102°F by rectum." Instead of saying "He has diarrhea", say, "He has had ten large watery bowel movements in the last six hours."

√ Be ready to give (1) the age and approximate weight of your child; (2) when he started to get sick; (3) if he has a fever and if so how much; (4) what you think is wrong with the child, other illnesses in the family, if any, and what you have done so far.

√ If your child has a cold or cough, be prepared to describe the cough (dry, loose, crowing, painful) and breathing (normal, fast, labored). Find out before your call if he has a headache, earache, sore throat, joint or chest pain.

√ If your child has a stomachache or pain, be ready to describe the location of the pain, how the child reacts to the pain, if the abdomen feels tight or rigid, if the child has been hit in the stomach, and if he has any other symptoms such as headache, nausea, or vomiting.

√ If your child has been injured, describe the details of the accident and your impression of his general condition (alert, dazed, listless, or unconscious).

When To Call Your Physician Immediately

You should call your physician at any hour of the day or night if your child has any of the following symptoms. (If you cannot reach your physician, call for an ambulance or take your child to the Hospital Emergency Room.)

√ Bleeding that cannot be stopped by direct pressure on the wound

√ Unconsciousness

√ Anything beyond a local skin reaction to an insect

sting or a recent injection if it occurs within 30 minutes, such as fever, bone joint pain, vomiting, headache, generalized hives and tightness in throat or chest.

√ Breathing dificulties: Your child is gasping, extremely anxious, or turning blue.

√ Convulsions: May be caused by high fever, infections, or epilepsy. Put the child on a bed or soft surface, keep his face down or to the side, wipe secretions from his mouth and nose and stay with him until the convulsion is over. Have someone call the physician as quickly as possible. Convulsions usually last only a few minutes. If they last longer, take your child to the hospital emergency room to be treated, if your physician cannot attend to him immediately.

√ Abdominal pain lasting more than an hour or two: Give the child nothing to eat or drink and do not give any laxative. Abdominal pain, especially when accompanied by fever and vomiting, could indicate appendicitis or other serious abdominal conditions.

√ Black, bloody, or tarry bowel movement in an infant who is not taking iron. This could indicate external (nose or mouth) or internal bleeding.

√ Diarrhea in infancy: If an infant has three or four loose watery stools, he could rapidly develop dehydration. Watch for signs of dehydration such as listlessness, fever, dry lips and skin, and failure to urinate.

When To Call Your Physician During Office Hours

You should call your physician during his regular office or phone hours for any of the symptoms listed below. You should also call if your child is acting sick, even if he doesn't have any specific complaints. (Some of the following conditions are described more fully in the text. See the Index.)

THE FIRST YEAR

√ *Vomiting:* Simple vomiting or spitting up in a young infant generally is not serious. But if vomited material spurts out one or two feet, it could indicate a serious intestinal problem, especially in infants under two months.

√ *Unusual crying:* Become familiar with your baby's normal cries and learn to distinguish unusual ones. Grunting or whining cries or hoarseness may mean trouble. Most newborns cry and fret between one and three hours per day. If you can find no apparent reason for continued crying, call your physician.

√ *Fever:* A temperature over 101°F (38.3°C) for two or more hours, as well as any symptoms that accompany it, should be reported to your physician.

PRESCHOOL AGE (1 TO 6)

√ *Fever:* A temperature over 101°F (38.3°C) for two or more hours as well as any symptoms that accompany it should be reported to your physician.

√ *Persistent headaches:* Like fever, headache is a symptom of many conditions, including allergy, fatigue, or infection. If a child complains of headache more than twice a week, or if the headache is associated with nausea or vomiting, consult your physician.

√ *Dizziness:* This may or may not be a symptom of something serious. If a child has been doing somersaults or running in circles, any immediate dizziness is natural.

However, if the child under normal circumstances is clumsy, cannot keep his balance or constantly feels dizzy, this may be serious and should be reported to your physician.

√ *Persistent vomiting* may mean intestinal obstruction, metabolic disease, a kidney problem, or other chronic disease—especially if associated with weight loss.

√ *Unusual fatigue and weight loss:* If fatigue persists for a number of days, is accompanied by weight loss, or is associated with an activity that has never before tired the child, it may be a sign of a number of illnesses that need to be investigated.

√ *Constant cough or hoarseness:* Even if it started with a head cold or flu, a nagging cough or hoarseness should be checked with your physician, especially if it keeps the child awake at night with loss of sleep and subsequent fatigue during the day.

√ *Frequent sore throats and mouth breathing* may indicate enlarged adenoids or tonsils.

√ *Frequent nosebleeds:* Children commonly have nosebleeds. If bleeding continues after simple first aid measures, such as constant pressure to the bleeding nostril for several minutes, consult your physician. Frequent bleeding of the nose at night or while the child is inactive may be a sign of a medical problem that needs attention.

√ *Sore or swollen joints:* A healthy, active child may occasionally complain of aching joints resulting from excessive physical activity. But for continued pain, swelling, redness, or lack of mobility the child should be examined by the physician, *especially if there is any fever.*

√ *Frequent or painful urination:* A change in urinary pattern may signal a medical problem. Frequent, painful urination (every half hour or so) or recurrence of bed-wetting may mean a urinary tract infection, especially in young girls. Frequent urination or recurrence of bedwetting may also be a sign of diabetes.

√ *Enlarged lymph nodes in neck and sore throat:* Lymph tissue is part of the body's defense system against infection. These glands may often be felt in children and do not necessarily mean anything is abnormal. Swollen glands are sometimes, however, associated with various infections — respiratory ailments, tonsillitis, German measles, mumps, and mononucleosis.

√ *Abdominal pain:* Any pain in the area below the ribs is a cause for concern, though not necessarily alarm. Swelling, tenderness, bloating, rigidity or increasing severity of pain may be symptoms of a serious condition.

√ *Croup* is a loud, deep, dry cough often coupled with breathing difficulties, characterized by a "crowing" sound on breathing in. You can help your child breathe by using a humidifier or you can get your bathroom steamed up by running the hot water in the shower. Stay with your child for half an hour or so. Be calm; try to show no fear or alarm. Croup with fever is more serious than croup without.

√ *Asthma* is a disorder in which the airway bronchial tubes narrow from time to time, causing the child to have difficulty in breathing. It is characterized by wheezing on breathing out. Asthma may be triggered by emotional factors or infection. A child having an asthma attack requires immediate treatment to relieve his bronchial spasms and long-range care to find the cause, if he does not respond to his regular asthma medication.

√ *Earache:* Earaches are common from infancy to six or seven years of age. Most, but not all, follow a stuffy nose and colds. If an infant rubs his ear or cries incessantly when he has a cold, especially at night, suspect an earache. Your physician should be called to treat the earache. Chronic ear infections can produce hearing loss.

√ *Skin changes:* If a skin cut, bruise, or rash doesn't heal in a few days, consult your physician to make sure there is no serious cause. Similarly, slow-healing cuts or bruises and continuing rashes or itching anywhere on the body should be reported.

EARLY SCHOOL AGE (6-9)

√ *Puffy eyes, swollen hands, and feet:* Not uncommonly, some children awaken each morning with puffy eyes caused by an allergy which should be reported to a physician and treated. But, more seriously, the child who has puffy eyes or swollen hands and cannot put on his shoes because of swollen feet may have signs of a kidney problem.

√ *Muscle weakness:* If a child was formerly active and can no longer go up and down stairs easily or run about without becoming weak, your physician should check for a possible neuromuscular problem.

√ *Bedwetting:* After the age of two, children generally have normal control. But repeated bedwetting in a child of six or more is a medical problem called *enuresis.* The child could have a urinary tract infection or abnormality or an emotional problem. Bedwetting in a child who previously had control could signify an infection or diabetes and should be checked by your physician.

√ *School phobia:* At the start of or during the school year, many children complain of ailments ranging from headache to upset stomach. If a child regularly complains of multiple ailments on school days which extend through the week-end, and asks to stay home from school, a physician should be consulted to determine whether there is an emotional problem or a physical disorder.

√ *Poor classroom performance:* If a child does poorly in school, he should be examined to determine whether there is a vision, hearing, learning or emotional problem.

What To Mention to Your Physician at Your Next Visit

You should discuss any changes in your child's emotional, social or physical behavior or what seems to you to be a delay in development with your physician during your next office visit. The following items are not cause for immediate concern, but should be checked.

THE FIRST YEAR

√ *Failure to notice moving objects:* At birth a baby cannot see clearly. If an infant over three months of age fails to respond to what is happening around him, this should be checked.

√ *Absence of leg kicks:* If you hold an infant upright under his arms, he will normally raise and lower his legs as if walking. Failure to do so may mean a nerve or muscle problem.

√ *Failure to hold his head up:* If a baby is unable to hold his head up by three months, roll over by four to five months, or sit up alone by eight months, consult a physician concerning a possible developmental problem.

√ *Failure to pull himself up or toddle:* After a baby starts to creep, he learns to pull himself up and attempt a few steps. If an infant of 10 to 14 months cannot do this, reasons may vary from a neurological disorder to malnutrition.

√ *Absence of teeth:* A baby's first teeth usually should appear between three and eight months but long delays are not unusual.

√ *A fat, flabby baby:* An overly fat baby is not necessarily a healthy baby. A baby who receives a diet that is essentially milk after 4-6 months with no solid food may have too large a proportion of fat to muscle. This can be corrected by a change in diet. However, poor muscle tone or flabbiness may also be a sign of an underlying medical problem.

√ *No attempt to mimic sounds or words:* Some babies utter their first word at five months; others, not until they are a year old or older. If a baby doesn't mimic sounds by one year, he should be seen by your physician.

PRESCHOOL AGE (1-6)

√ *Unusual or excessive activity:* A healthy, active child is inquisitive and venturesome. But a child who is continually restless and overactive may be evidencing hyperkinetic behavior. Other signs are short attention span in school and clumsiness. Such problem children are usually normal mentally. Hyperkinetic behavior can often be controlled after it is evaluated.

√ *Poor muscle coordination:* Many children go through an awkward phase, occasionally falling while running or skipping. But unusual clumsiness or unexpected chronic awkwardness could be a symptom of some potentially serious disorder.

What To Expect at the Hospital Emergency Room

Emergency rooms in medical facilities are busy places. They are organized for dealing with life-threatening situations in the most efficient way possible. Know where the nearest emergency facility is, how to get there (whether by ambulance or by your car), and about how long a ride it will take. Expect:

√ To wait in a separate area for an extended period of time. Diagnosis and treatments are often long delayed. Make arrangements before you leave with someone to babysit for any other children left at home while you are gone.

√ To sign releases for necessary treatment. These are legal requirements which all medical facilities must carry out.

√ To complete and sign papers which describe how the medical facility will be paid for the care it gives. This also includes the ambulance service, which often is privately owned. Bring along your checkbook, health-care cards (such as Blue Cross) or certificates, and as much cash as is available. Know your Social Security Number.

√ To consult with the professional staff about the treatment your child is to receive once he is stabilized and all life support measures have been taken. You should feel free, and insist if necessary, to consult with the doctor of your choice if special or continuing procedures will be needed.

√ Know the name and telephone number of the doctor who is to be consulted, and who may admit the child to the hospital under his service.

Home First Aid Gear

All first aid supplies should be quickly accessible. Keep them in a "first aid" container, labeled so. Children in the family should be taught to leave these materials alone except when instructed by an adult to use them. Quantities should be limited to what will be useful for one or two occasions and, when used up, should be replaced promptly.

The following items should be in every home first aid kit where there are children:

√ Syrup of Ipecac—one ounce bottle
√ Activated charcoal—small can
√ Fever thermometers (rectal and mouth)
√ Sterile gauze compresses—6 to 12 in 3- or 4-inch sizes
√ Adhesive tape
√ Adhesive strip bandages with gauze pads
√ Antiseptic or antibiotic cream or ointment
√ One gallon of sterile or distilled water (handy to kit; once opened, do not keep for a long period)
√ Tweezers, safety pins, small and large scissors, needles
√ Flashlight, extra batteries
√ Absorbent cotton, roll of elastic bandage
√ Petroleum jelly
√ Baking soda (bicarbonate of soda)
√ Rubbing alcohol
√ An icebag and a hot water bag
√ A small bottle of aromatic spirits of ammonia
√ A supply of dry matches
√ A box of sterile cotton-tipped applicators
√ A clean cloth at least 40 inches by 40 inches square, to make a triangular bandage
√ A bottle of aspirin
√ Two wood splints about one foot long and three inches wide; a supply of tongue depressors for finger splinting

Dressings and Bandages

Application of a protective covering to wounds and burns helps prevent the entry of dirt and germs and can thus do much to reduce the possibility of infection. It also has a psychological value, since it conceals the injury and tends to lessen the injured child's anxieties and fears. The ideal covering consists of an inner *dressing* or compress which comes directly in contact with the wound, and an outer *bandage* which holds the dressing in place. Since the dressing actually touches an injury, it must not only be clean but also free of germs (sterile). Gauze is the best for first aid dressings, since it is highly absorbent and at the same time porous enough to admit some air to the wound while providing excellent protection.

Most home and family emergency situations requiring bandaging can be met with the following types of bandages:

√ triangular bandage (e.g., arm sling)
√ cravat bandage (e.g., ankle sprain)
√ butterfly bandage

Triangular Bandages

The triangular bandage is made from a square of material about 40 × 40 inches. Use muslin, but a clean bed sheet will do. Cut the square from corner to corner, and you have two triangular bandages. ("A" in illustrations).

The triangular bandage can be used for many purposes—for supporting the arm in a sling, and for covering injuries of the chest, back, shoulder, face, head, upper arm, thigh, hand, or foot where a fairly large area must be bandaged.

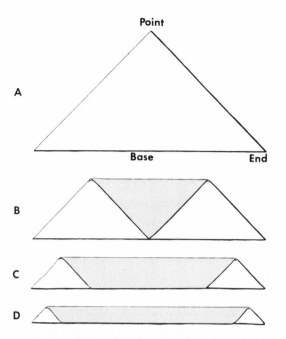

Folding a triangular bandage to make a cravat bandage.

Cravat Bandages

In some cases, the triangular bandage is more effective if it is folded before use since folding gives added strength. In its folded form, the triangular bandage is called a cravat bandage and looks something like a necktie or cravat as illustrated ("C" and "D"). Such a bandage can be used to apply firm pressure for the control of bleeding and to give support for a sprained ankle, for example. Folding also adapts the bandage better to such hard-to-bandage spots as the elbow, knee and head.

To prepare the cravat bandage, spread a triangular bandage out flat. Fold over the point to the base as shown in (B). Then fold the bandage lengthwise one or more times ("C" and "D") until the desired width is obtained. This type of bandage can be used to hold dressings in place on the head, cheek, ear, eye, neck, thigh, leg, upper arm, palm, elbow, and knee. In each instance, the dressing is held in place with the fingers, and the cravat is wrapped around the part, adjusted to its contours, and tied at its ends with a square knot.

The cravat bandage made from a triangular bandage is useful for emergency binding of a sprained ankle.

"Butterfly" Bandage (strips)

When a wound or laceration is not too large or deep, the edges can be held in place with so-called "butterfly" strips. These are available in any drugstore, ready made and sterilized. If, however, these are not readily available in the home at the time of an accident, strips can easily be made by a simple procedure shown in the illustrations below. These strips are applied in such a way as to draw the edges of the wound together, thus helping to control bleeding and aiding the skin edges to grow together without the use of sutures (stitches). This technique is time (and money) saving, easily applied, painless and is particularly useful with children and apprehensive adults. If done properly, scarring would not be any more noticeable than with stitches.

Temperature-Pulse-Respiration (TPR): Method

The body temperature, pulse, and respiration rate provide a valuable index to your child's state of health. They serve as a guide to the seriousness of an illness and the progress being made in overcoming any disease or injury.

You cannot rely on the "TPR" as an infallible guide, however, since your child may be ill and still have only

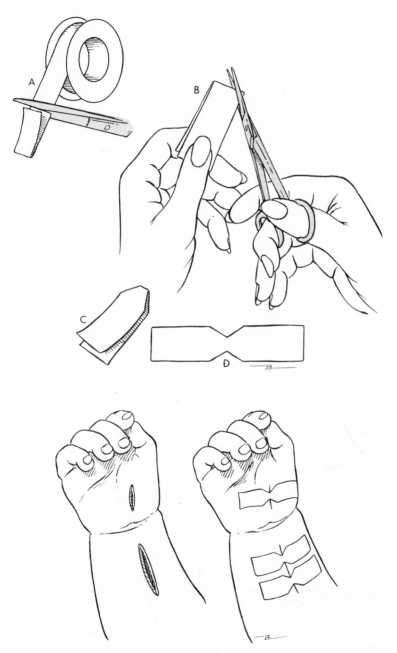

Making and applying a "butterfly" bandage.

slightly abnormal temperature, pulse, and respiration. In some instances, the temperature may be quite high even in a moderate illness. In spite of these exceptions, the information about temperature, pulse, and respiration is important for you and your physician to know when you call him.

Temperature Taking

A sick child should have his temperature taken morning and night (every four hours if it is high, unless a physician directs otherwise). If the temperature shows any large change from the last time it was taken, check the reading again. If the difference is confirmed, notify the physician. Pulse and respiration are usually counted at the same time the temperature is taken.

Kinds of Thermometers. Temperature can be taken by mouth or by rectum. Oral (mouth) thermometers differ in appearance from that of the rectal thermometer (see illustration). Temperature can also be taken by placing the oral thermometer in the armpit, but this method is not recommended, since readings can be inaccurate unless taken over a period of five minutes or more.

Reading a Thermometer. Thermometers may come in gradations reading in the Fahrenheit (F°) scale or the Celsius (C°) scale. At the top of the accompanying illustration, a quick comparison between normal and high temperatures between these two scales is given.

To convert Fahrenheit readings to Celsius, read the Fahrenheit scale, subtract 32, multiply by 5, and divide by 9.

Example: 98.6°F − 32 = 66.6
times 5 = 333
divided by 9 = 37°C

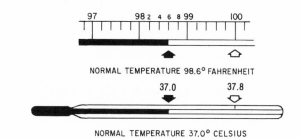

NORMAL TEMPERATURE 98.6° FAHRENHEIT

37.0   37.8

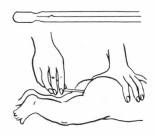

NORMAL TEMPERATURE 37.0° CELSIUS

| *Taking a temperature by mouth.* | *Taking a temperature by rectum.* |

To reverse the procedure, that is, to convert Celsius to Fahrenheit, read the Celsius scale, divide by 5, multiply by 9, and add 32.

Example: 37°C divided by 5 = 7.4

times 9 = 66.6

add 32 = 98.6°F

Hold the thermometer by its top, as shown. Note that the glass tube, which contains mercury, may be triangular or round in shape. On most thermometers, one side of the triangle is marked off in gradations; the second side bears a row of figures ranging from 92°F upwards, or equivalent Celsius figures; the third side has a broad white or colored line. Hold the thermometer in a good light so that the point of the triangle made by the gradation side and the figure side is toward you. Now slowly turn the thermometer back and forth between the thumb and index finger until you locate the silvery looking column of mercury. The triangular shape of the thermometer magnifies this to the nearest gradation of the scale.

If the thermometer is round instead of triangular, turn the thermometer until the column of mercury and scale are visible, hold to a good light, and read.

Shaking Down a Thermometer. Always shake down the column of mercury in a thermometer before taking a temperature; it doesn't go down automatically. Grasp the thermometer firmly between thumb and index finger and give a downward shake with a vigorous snapping action, but be sure to hold the thermometer tightly. Read the thermometer and if the reading is above 95°F (or 35°C) repeat the shaking until the mercury reaches that point or below.

Taking Temperature by Mouth. This is the usual method of taking temperature unless the child is unconscious, uncontrollable, or for some reason unable to hold his mouth tightly closed—he may be unable to breathe through his nose, for example.

Clean the thermometer with a small piece of cotton or a bit of paper tissue which has been wet in *cool* water, and then soaped slightly. Pull the thermometer back and forth through the cotton with a turning motion so that it is thoroughly cleaned. Then rinse the thermometer in clear, cool water. (Do *not* use hot water; it will break the thermometer.) Shake down the thermometer as described above.

Have your child lie down or sit. Ask him to open his mouth, and gently place the thermometer under the tongue on one side. He should then close his lips tightly around the thermometer, *but not clamp down on it with his teeth*. Leave the thermometer in this position for about three minutes.

Remove the thermometer, wipe with dry cotton or tissue, and read the temperature as described above. Average or "normal" mouth temperature is 98.6° Fahrenheit (37° Celsius.) However, for a particular individual "normal" may be a bit lower or higher.

After the temperature has been read, clean the thermometer again as described above, rinse in cool water, wipe dry with clean cotton or tissue, and replace in its case.

Taking the Temperature by Rectum. This is the usual method of taking temperature in a baby or small child, or an unconscious older child. Clean the rectal thermometer and shake it down as described above. Lubricate it with petroleum jelly or mineral oil. If a rectal thermometer is not available, an oral thermometer can be used in the same manner, if care is taken and the child can be controlled.

Have the child lie on his side if possible. Then gently insert the thick bulb end of the thermometer about an inch into the rectum. Hold the thermometer in this position with the fingers for about three minutes, counting the time by a watch or clock.

Be very careful in using rectal thermometers in uncooperative children. Hold the thermometer firmly, and be prepared to remove it quickly if your child thrashes about suddenly. There is danger that he will break the tube and injure himself.

Remove the thermometer carefully, wipe it off with dry cotton or tissue, and read the temperature. Average or "normal" rectal temperature is higher than normal mouth temperature—that is, 99.6° Fahrenheit or 37.5° Celsius. Keep this in mind, since the "normal" point as indicated by an arrow on the thermometer will show 98.6° Fahrenheit (37° Celsius). Clean the thermometer as described above and return it to its case.

Guarding Against Error. Mouth temperature should

not be taken for half an hour after your child has had a hot or cold drink or has chewed gum. Rectal temperature should not be taken for half an hour after the child has had a hot or cold tub bath. Otherwise, the reading may not be correct. Expect elevation of temperature after vigorous activity or exercise.

Pulse Counting

Pulse is best counted at the wrist, where the radial artery lies close to the surface, but if the wrists are injured, pulse can be counted at the temple or even at the ankle.

Place the first three fingers of your hand on the inner surface of the wrist just below the child's thumb as shown. Press down gently, but firmly, with the fingertips until artery pulsations can easily be felt. Now count the pulsations that occur in a half-minute period, using a watch with a second hand for timing. Wait a few seconds and then repeat the count for another half-minute period. The two figures should be almost identical. If there is a difference of more than one or two between the counts, repeat the procedure. Then add the two counts together for the pulse rate, which is customarily expressed in pulsations per minute.

The average pulse rate in an older child is about 70 to 80 per minute when he is at rest. Variations are common, however; some people have a normal pulse rate of about 60, others one of 90. The pulse rate also tends to vary with age. In babies, the pulse rate may range from 120 to 130 per minute. The pulse rate increases with exercise and emotion, and usually with fever and illness. Like the temperature, it is a valuable sign of the body's condition.

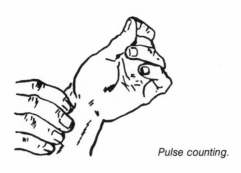

Pulse counting.

Respiratory Count

The rate and rhythm of respirations are usually counted at the same time the temperature is taken and pulse counted. It is always best not to let your child realize that his breathing is being checked, since it is easy to vary rate or rhythm, and he may do so unintentionally if he becomes self-conscious. Let your fingers remain on the child's wrist for an extra minute after the pulse has been taken. During this minute, the respirations are counted.

Each respiration consists of a complete breathing cycle, one rise of the chest wall (inspiration) and one fall of the chest wall (expiration). Older children usually have 15 to 20 respirations per minute when at rest; younger children, 20 to 25; and babies, 30 to 35. Respirations tend to increase with exercise and emotion, and with the pulse rate and temperature. An illness in the chest, such as pneumonia, causes respirations to increase at a much greater rate proportionately than do the pulse and temperature.

Immunization Record

Recently, some increases have been noted in childhood diseases, such as polio and measles, which seem to be the result of negligence in getting immunizations for a child at the prescribed time and frequency.

It is vital that you take your child to the physician or health care center at the following suggested ages for his immunizations against these preventable diseases: diphtheria, tetanus, pertussis (whooping cough), polio, measles, rubella (German measles) and mumps. Ask your doctor to make a record of the date of immunization on this page so that you'll know what immunizations your child has had.

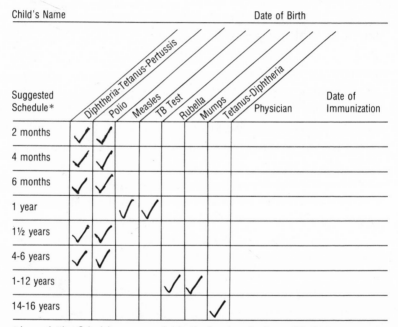

Child's Name _____ Date of Birth _____

Suggested Schedule*	Diphtheria-Tetanus-Pertussis	Polio	Measles	TB Test	Rubella	Mumps	Tetanus-Diphtheria	Physician	Date of Immunization
2 months	✓	✓							
4 months	✓	✓							
6 months	✓	✓							
1 year			✓	✓					
1½ years	✓	✓							
4-6 years	✓	✓							
1-12 years					✓	✓			
14-16 years							✓		

* Immunization Schedule recommended by the American Academy of Pediatrics

INDEX

tantrums and, 211-2
Breathing, 212
  absence of, 212
  death and, 212
  epiglottitis and, 215
  failure of, 176-7
  fast, 212
  irregular, 212
  mouth, 247
  problems, 41
    physician for, 245
Brews, 83
Bribing child, 72
Broad jump, 45
Brooks, 48
Broth, heating, 79
Bruises, 220-1
  coloration, 220
  fracture and, 221
  lacerations and, 188
  minor, 220
  severe, 220
  slow-healing, 249
  treatment, 221-2
  unexplained, 220-1
Bubble bath, ingestion, 75
Bubble-blowing exercise, 49
Bug spray, see Insecticides
Building inspection department, 112
Bulbs, plant, 90-1
Burns, 26, 43
  area covered, 180-1
  bandage for, 181-2
  chemical, 182-3
  clothing removal, 181
  cold-water treatment, 181-2
  degree of, 180-1
  electric, 183-4
  eye, 182-3
  grease application, 179
  heat, 181-2
  lightning, 183
  prevention, 47
  shock and, 180
  treatment, 179-84

Bus drivers, 130-1
  distraction of, 59
Buses, 58-9, 130-2
  school, 129-32
    adult monitors on, 131-2
    drivers, 130-1
    safety standards, 131
    seat belts, 131
    waiting area, 129
Buttercup, 90, 92
Butterfly bandage, see Bandages, butterfly
Butterfly strip, 256-7
Buttons, 33

Cabinets, 17
Caladium, 92
Calamine lotion, hives and, 231-2
Calf (leg), protrusion, 202
Calla lily, 90
Campers, 76
Campfires, 121
Camping, 119-22
  necessities for, 119-20
  safety rules, 120
Camps, 122-3
  accident occurrence, 122
  supervision, 122
Candles, 150
  fire hazard, 148
  ingestion, 75
Candy, from strangers, 136
  hard, 51
  medicine and, 37, 72
Canning, commercial, 181
Canning, home, 81
Cans, bulging, 81
Caps, toy pistol, ingestion, 75
Car pools, 16
Car seats, 95-7
  installation, 98-9
Car shield, 56
Carbon monoxide, 75-6
Carbonated beverages, vomiting induction and, 175

Extension cords, 144
Extension plugs, 143
Eye
  black, 190, 220
  chemical burn, 182-3
    flushing after, 812-3
  drug use and, 216
  glasses and, 142
  imbedded object, 203
  infant movement of, 250
  injuries, 142
  oil for, 203
  particle removal, 203-4
  puffy, 249
  pupil size variation, 199
  washing solution, 203
Eyeglasses, 142-3

Fabric, flammable, see Clothing, flammable
Factory Mutual Label, 111
Fahrenheit to Celsius conversion, 258-9
Fainting, 173-4, 213
Falls, 27-8
  home, 157
  infant, 27-8
  prevention, 27-8
Family
  changes in, 155
  problems, 60-1
Fans, 39, 113
Farm equipment, see Tractors, farm
Fatigue
  accidents and, 7
  drug use and, 216
  unusual, 247
Feces eating, 35
Feeding, infant, 27, 36, 40
Feet
  flat, 202
  swollen, 249
Fences, 18
Fever, 246
  cause of, 212

convulsions and, 210-1
reduction of, 210-1
reportable, 246
swollen joints and, 247
Fighting, 126
  protection from, 129
Finger, dislocation, 200
  fracture, 195
Finger paints, 139
Fingernail, blackened, 222
  saving, 222
Fingertip, bruised, 222
Fire alarms, 110-1
Fire department, calling 106-7
  handicapped and, 62-3
Fire drills, 108-9, 133
Fire extinguishers, 110-1
Fire salts, 150
Firearms, see Guns
Fireplaces, 34, 158
Fires, 62-3
  clothing, 109-10
  electrical, 111-2
  escape routes, 108-9
  evacuation, 108-9
  grease, 111
  handicapped and, 62-3
Fireworks, 151-2
First aid, 185-6, 289-92
  accident chart, 289-91
  guidelines, 167-8
  kit contents, 253-6
  poisoning chart, 292
  professional help and, 167-8
    sources of, 94
  training, 165
  see also names of specific injuries
Fishbowl agents, ingestion, 75
Fishhook accidents, 223-4
Flammable liquids, 112
Flashlight
  batteries, ingestion, 75
  need for, 112
Floating, 49-50
  drownproofing technique, 106-7

cause of, 232
first-aid, 232
infants and, 232
Highchair, 30
location of, 34, 47
Highway, walking on, 129
Hiking, 118-22
Hives, 245
appearance of, 231
avoidance, 231
treatment, 231-2
Hoarseness, 247
Hobby equipment, 138-9
Holly berries, 150
Home, child-oriented, 236-7
other people's, 17
Hopping, ability, 45
Hoses, 110
Hospital emergency room, *see* Emergency room
"Hot", use of, 47
Hot applications, 207
Hot materials, 47
House wiring, 143-4
Household cleaners, *see* Cleaning agents
Houses, empty, 135
Human bites, 193
infection hazard, 193
Hunger, accidents and, 7
Hunting, 115
Hyacinths, 82, 90, 93
Hyoscyamine, 216
Hyperactivity, 7, 251
Hyperkinetic behavior, 251
Hypothermia, 120

Ice bag, bruises and, 221
sprains and, 207
Ice chests, hazards, 52
Illness, mother's, 7
sudden, 212-3
Imagination, period of, 46
Immunizations, record of, 263-4
schedule for, 264

Incisions, treatment, 187-8
Infant, 4, 246, 250
age groups
0-4 months, 26-31
4-7 months, 31-37
7-12 months, 38-40
diet, 251
fat, 251
feeding, 27, 36, 40
flabby, 251
food preservation for, 36
head support, 26, 30
leaving alone, 27
pulling self up, 250-1
rescue breathing technique, 169-72
safety rules, 26
siblings and, 30-1
sight in, 250
sound imitation by, 251
sudden death, 40-41
symptoms to report, 250-1
toys for, 30-1, 34, 138
Infants, newborn, 26-31
capabilities, 25
development, 26-7
falls, 27-8
feeding, 27
safety rules, 26
toys for, 30-1, 138
Infant seat, 32
Infectious hepatitis, pets and, 145
Injury, categories of, 166
moving after 185-6
Inkberry, 91, 92
Insect bites, 226-8
allergy and, 226
kits for, 226
physician for, 244-5
treatment, 226
Insect repellant, 119
Insecticides, 39
ingestion, 75
storage, 72
substitutes for, 89
see also Pesticides

Insomnia, drug use and, 216
Interchange, learning through, 12-4
International Association for Medical Assistance to Travelers, 242
International Guild for Infant Survival, 41
Intersections, 128
  bicycles and, 142
Intestinal flu, appendicitis and, 234
Intoxication, 217
Ipecac syrup, 253
  dosage, 175, 214
Irons, 113, 158
Irrigation ditches, 135
Isolation temporary, as discipline, 19
Isopropyl alcohol, 217
Itchiness, 249
Ivy, poison, 86

Jars, baby food, 36, 39
Jessamine, 90
  carolinas, 92
  yellow, 92
Jimsonweed, 90, 92, 216
Joints, discoloration around, 206
  dislocated, 200-1
  fever plus pain in, 247
  painful, 202, 206, 247
  sprained, 205-7
  see also names of specific joints
Jonquil, 91
Judgment, age and, 17-8
  child's, 17-8
Junk yard, 135

Kerosene, 175
  ingestion, 75
Kiddy cars, as toys, 139
Kidney problem, symptom of, 249
Kitchen, 34
  barricades, 34
  cabinets, 17
  child in, 34
  range, 158

Kites, age for, 139
  construction, 123
  flying, 123
  lightning and, 123
  power lines and, 123
Knee sprain, 206
Kwell, preparation for lice, 229

Labels, 36-7
Laceration, 188-9
  cleaning, 188
  non-suture closing, 189
Ladders, fire, 109
  playground, 134
  pool, 104
Ladybug, as insect control, 89
Lamps, 39, 148
Lakes, 48, 51
Language, 10
Lantana, 92
Lap belts, 95-6
Larkspur, 90, 93
Latches, safety, 53
Laughing jags, drug use and, 216
Laundry products, 74-5
Laurel, 90, 92
Lawn mowers, 116-8
  blade speed, 117
  engine exhaust, 117
  handles, 117
  overturning, 116
  pets and, 117
  refuelling, 118
  safety features, 116-7
Lead, pencil, ingestion, 75
Lead poisoning, 76-7
Leaf, lobed, 86
  toothed, 86
Learning, 10
  methods, 12-21
  observation and, 12
Leaves, as poisons, 82, 90, 91
Leftovers, 79, 80
Leg cramps, 202
Leg kick, failure to, 250

Lenses, safety, 142-3
Leptospirosis, pets and, 145
Lice, 228-9
 occurrence, 228
 elimination of, 228-9
Life style, 8-9
Lifeguards, 105
Light, traffic safety and, 143, 151
Light bulb changing, 144
Lighter fluid, ingestion, 75
Lightning, 50, 121
 burn pattern, 183
 defensive posture, 121
 kites and, 123
 swimming and, 50
Lily-of-the-valley, 91, 93
Liquids, flammable, 112, 159
 hot, 34, 39
Liquor, *see* Alcohol drinking; Alcoholism, parental
Live wire, rescue from, 177, 184
Locust tree, 90, 92
Love, carefulness and, 9
LSD, 216
Lymph nodes, enlarged, 248

Macaroni salad, 80
Maple pollen, 85
Marbles, 31
Marihuana, odor of, 216
 symptoms of use, 216
Marsh marigold, 90, 92
Masks, Halloween, 150
 mouth, making of, 181
Matches, 108, 159
Mattress, firmness, 31
 infant, 31
 straps for, 28-9
Measles, immunization, 264
Meat, cold, 80
 cooking, 80
 leftover, 79-80
 refrigeration, 80
 thawing frozen, 78
Mechanical hazards, *see* Hazards,

mechanical
Medicine cabinets, 71
Medical schools, 64, 94
Medicines, 71-2
 administering, 72
 candy-flavored, 37
 disposal of, 71
 dosage, 37
 home-made, 83
 interchanging use of, 72
 labels, 71
 storage, 71
 travel and, 242
Menstruation, mother's, 7, 155
Mercury, ingestion, 75
Metal cleaner, ingestion, 74
Metal polish, ingestion, 74
Methanol, 217
Microscopes, as toys, 139
Milk, inhalation by infant, 27
 refrigeration, 36
Minibike, 100-2
 accidents with, 101-2
 helmet use, 101
 licensing, 101
 power range, 100
 protective clothing, 101
 wire hazard, 101-2
Mining areas, 135
Mistakes, child's, 56
Mistletoe, 91, 93
Mobiles, 138
Modeling kits, 139
Molesters, 129-30, 136
Monkshood, 90, 93
Mononucleosis, 248
Morphine, 216
Mother's health, accidents, and 7-8
Mother's lap, as car seat, 98
Motivation, 10-1
Motor boats, 51
Motor vehicles, accidents, 43, 47
 see also Automobiles; Minibike
 Motorcyles
Motorcycles, 102

Poisons, 35-7
  packaging, 89
  storage, 36, 53
  swallowed, 174-6
  see also names of specific poisons
Pokeberry, 91
Pokeweed, 91, 92
Polio immunization, 264
Pollens, 83, 87
Ponds, 48, 51
Pools, *see* Swimming pools
Popcorn, 39, 51
Poplar pollen, 85
Pot handles, 47
Potholes, 102
Potato salad, 80
Poultry, 77, 78, 79
Power lines, 123
Power mowers, *see* Lawn mowers
Pre-school child, training, 13-4
Precatory bean, 93
Pregnancy, mother's, as stress factor,
  7, 155
Prescriptions, 71-2; *see also* Drugs;
  Medicines
Pressure points, 174
Products, hazardous, 19, 67-8
  See also names of specific products
Projectiles, 137
  toys and, 138
Propellants, aerosol, 74
Protection, definition, 4
Psychosis, drug use and, 216
Puppets, as toys, 139
Pulse, 243
  average, 262
  counting method, 262
  rate,
    child's, 262
    infant's, 262
  significance of, 262
  variation in, 262
Pumpkin, candle-lit, 150
Puncture wounds, 189-90
  bleeding and, 190

causes of, 189
cleaning, 189
infection, 190
internal damage, 190
Punishment, 13-4, 19
Pupil (eye) size, drug use and, 216
  variation in, 199
Pups, cautions for, 146
Putty, 76
Puzzles, as toys, 45

Rabbit fever, 227
Rabies, occurrence, 193
  pets and, 145
  treatment, 193
Radiators, 159
  covers for, 34
Ragweed, 84, 85, 87
Railroad property, hazards, 135
Rain, hazards of, 121
Ramps, use of, 62
Rash, 249
Rat poison, ingestion, 75
Rattles, 30, 139
Reach, infant ability, 31
  safety and, 69
Ready Reference Guide, 240-64
Reason, learning to, 17
Reassurance, shock and, 173
Rebellions, 46, 215
Recreation programs, 133-5
Rectal temperature, taking, 261-2
Red Cross, 104
Reflective tape, use of, 143, 150
Refrigeration, 76-9
Refrigerators, 51-2
  abandoned, 52
  safety measures, 51-2
  suffocation in, 52
  temperature of, 78
Regulation, definition, 4
Rehabilitation care, 63
Rehabilitation center, 64
Releases for treatment, signing, 252
Reprimands, 18

pets and, 228
protective clothing for, 228
removal, 227-8
repellants, 228
Tinsel, lead containing, 150
Toddlers, 44-7
infants and, 31
restrictions for, 17
teaching of, 46-7
Toilet, use of, 43
Tongue, removal from airway, 169
Tonsillitis, 248
Tonsils, enlarged, 247
Tools, electric, 158
hand, as toys, 139
use of, 19, 57
Tooth, *see* Teeth
Tooth paste, ingestion, 75
Toothache, 232-3
first-aid, 233
Toxicity, meaning of, 88
Toxicodendron radicans, 86
Toxicodendron vernix, 87
Toys, 53-5, 137-9
age and, 138-9
4-7 months, 34, 138
7-12 months, 39-40, 43-5, 138
infants, 30-31, 138
dangerous, 7-8, 13
edges, 30
hanging, 30
in car, 99
inexpensive, 40
information on, 54-5
labels, 137
painted, 76
safe, 34, 53-5
selection guides, 53-5, 138-9
size, 42
squeeze, 34
suitability, 137-8
TPR method, 256-8
Tractors, brakes, 118
farm, 118
overturning, 118

Traffic hazards, age and, 124-5
Traffic light, 129
Traffic safety, 58, 124-5
playground vicinity, 133-4
school programs, 127-33
Trailers, 76
Trails, 101
Trains, electric, as toys, 139
Tranquilizers, suicide and, 218
Traveling
abroad, 242
child alone, 58
medications for, 242
physician access during, 242
school routes, 127-33
Treats, Halloween, 150
Trees, deciduous, 85; *see also* names
of specific trees
Triangular bandage, *see* Bandages,
triangular
Trick-or-treat, 150-1
accompanying child, 150
Tricycles, 140-1
accident factors, 140
double-riding, 140
repairs, 140-1
selection, 140
Tuberculosis test, 264
Tubs, water, 39
Tularemia, 227
Tuna salad, 80
Turning blue,
convulsions and, 209, 211
croup and, 214
epiglottitis and, 215
physician for, 245

Unconsciousness, 213
physician for, 244
vomiting induction and, 174
Undercooking, 81
Undertow, 105
Underwriters' Laboratories, Inc., 54
label, 112-3

Undress, ability to, 45
U.S. Consumer Product Safety Commission, 161
  hotline, 161
U.S. Department of Agriculture, 77
U.S. Food and Drug Administration, 77, 81
"Up" pills, 216
Urban areas, parent patrols, 130
Urinary tract infection, 248, 249
Urination,
  cessation, 245
  frequent, 247-8
  painful, 247-8
  pattern change, 247
Urticaria, *see* Hives
Use of things, safe, 19-21

Vacation time, accidents and, 8
Vaccination, *see* Immunization
Values, safety and, 9-10
Vaporizers, 39, 113
  bathroom use, 214
  cold air, 214
  croup and, 214
Vapors, flammable, 112-3
Varnishes, ingestion, 75
Vegetables, unwashed, 82
Venetian blinds, 32
Ventilation, 75-6
  baby's room, 40
  vehicles, 75-6
Visitors, strange, 136
Vitamins
  candy-flavored, 37
  dosage, 37
  storage, 37
Vomiting, 234, 246
  blood, 213
  causes, 213
  drugs and, 216
  head injury and, 199
  head position, 176
  inducement, 175-6
    avoiding of, 174

persistent, 247
spurting, 246

Wading pools, 135
Walking
  failure to, 251
  in traffic, 58, 129
  strangers and, 136
  unsteady, 200
Wallpaper, 76
Warnings, 13-4
Washers, 144-5; *see also* Wringers
Water
  distilled, 253
  fear of, 48
  hot, as hazard, 158-9
  safe age for play, 48
  scalding, 179
  shallow, 48; *See also* Water hazards
Water bodies, frozen, 48
Water games, 105
Water hazards, 48-51, 105, 135
  banks, steep, 51
  self-rescue, 105-7
Water-survival techniques, 106-7
Weather, cold, 229-30
  hazards, 120-1
  hot, 230-1
Weight loss, 247
Wells, 48
Wheals, 231
Whiplash, 197
Wheelchairs, safeguards for, 62
Whirlpools, 105
Whooping cough, immunization for 264
Wilderness survival, 119-22
Windows, 45
  non-breakable glass, 68
  tailgate, 76
Windpipe, blocked, 177-8
  clearing of, 177-8
Wiring, house, 158
  checking of, 112

First Aid

EMERGENCY TELEPHONE NUMBERS

Doctor	Ambulance/ Rescue Squad
Hospital	Poison Control Center
Dentist	Neighbor
Pharmacist	
Police	
Fire Dept.	

Pages 241-252

In Case of Serious Injury or Illness:
- Call a doctor, a hospital, the police or other emergency service **immediately.**
- Keep calm, briefly explain what has happened and ask what to do until help arrives.

First Aid Treatment:
- If you cannot get immediate help, the following safe measures may provide emergency relief.
- Refer to the pages of the book (listed in the left margin) for detailed information and guidance.

BLEEDING (SEVERE)

Pages 172-173

- Call for emergency help and transport to a medical facility.
- Do not use any antiseptics or other materials.
- Place a thick pad of clean cloth or bandage directly over wound and press firmly to control blood flow.
- Hold in place with strong bandage, neckties, cloth strips etc.
- Do not make tie so tight as to prevent circulation to the rest of the limb.
- In case of injuries to the groin, armpit or neck, where ties cannot be used, control blood flow with finger or hand pressure.
- Raise the bleeding part higher than the rest of the body, unless bones are broken.
- If injury is extensive, treat for shock (see below).

Nosebleeds

Pages 225-226

- Have patient in sitting position blow out from the nose all clot and blood.
- Insert into the bleeding nostril a wedge of cotton moistened with any of the common nose drops.
- With the finger against the outside of that nostril apply firm pressure for five minutes.
- If bleeding stops remove packing (no rush, here).
- Check with your doctor if bleeding persists.

BROKEN BONES

If a fracture of any part of the body or any injury to the head, neck or back is suspected, the patient should not be moved without medical supervision unless absolutely necessary.

If a patient with a back or neck injury must be moved, keep the back, head and neck in a straight line, preventing them from being twisted or bent during movement. Use a board to help keep back, neck and head rigid.

For other fractures, until you get medical help, place the injured part in as natural a position as possible without causing discomfort to the patient. Protect from further injury by applying splints long enough to extend well beyond the joints above and below the fracture. Any firm material can be used (board, pole, metal rod, or even a thick magazine or thick folded newspaper). Pad splints with clothing or other soft material to prevent skin injury. Fasten splints with bandage or cloth at the break and beyond joints above and below it. Use pressure bandage to control bleeding (see Bleeding).

Pages 194-199

BURNS AND SCALDS

- Get patient to doctor or hospital as soon as possible.
- If he is conscious and can swallow, give plenty of water or other non-alcoholic liquids to drink.
- Do not use ointments, greases, powders, etc.
- Until you get medical help, immerse burned area immediately in cold water or apply clean, cold, moist towels.
- Chill water with ice, if possible, *but never add salt.*
- Maintain treatment as long as pain or burning exists. In case of **chemical** burns, flush skin with plenty of running water.
- Cover burned area with clean cloth to exclude air.
- Avoid breaking any blisters that may appear.
- If burns are extensive keep patient quiet and treat for shock (see below).

Pages 179-184

CHOKING

- Use Heimlich maneuver as described on page 178. (Learn this technique as soon as possible.)
- If you cannot hold the child, have him lie on his back.
- Kneel over the child.
- Press crossed hands firmly against stomach above navel.
- Have someone ready to reach in mouth and remove food or other object.
- If the child cannot breathe at all, turn his head and face down over your knees and hit sharply between shoulder blades.

Pages 177-179

CONVULSIONS

- If caused by fever, sponge body with cool water.
- Apply cold cloths to head.
- Lay on side with hips elevated.
- Prevent biting of tongue.
- Be sure tongue is not blocking passage of air to the lung.
- Call physician.

Pages 208-211

EYE CONTAMINATION

Pages
182-183

- Remove contact lenses if worn; *never* permit the eye to be rubbed.
- Gently wash eye out immediately, using plenty of water (or milk in an emergency), for five minutes with eyelids held open.
- Call for emergency help and transport to a medical facility promptly.

FAINTING

Pages
173-174

- Keep in flat position.
- Elevate legs and feet.
- Loosen clothing around neck.
- Keep patient warm.
- Keep mouth clear.
- Give nothing to swallow.
- If breathing has stopped, start Artificial Respiration.
- Have someone call for emergency help and transport to a medical facility.

SHOCK

Pages
172-173

Shock usually accompanies severe injury or emotional upset. The signs are cold and clammy skin, pale face, chills, frequently nausea or vomiting, shallow breathing.

- Call for emergency help and treatment.
- Until you get medical help, have patient lie down with legs elevated.
- Keep patient covered to prevent chilling or loss of body heat.
- Give non-alcoholic fluids if he is able to swallow unless abdominal injury is suspected.

ARTIFICIAL RESPIRATION

Pages
169-171

There is need for help in breathing when breathing movements stop or lips, tongue, and fingernails become blue. When in doubt, apply artificial respiration until you get medical help. No harm can result from its use and delay may cost the patient his life. Start immediately. Seconds count.

- Clear mouth and throat of obstructions with your fingers.
- Place patient on back with face up.
- Lift the neck, tilt head back.
- If air passage is still closed, pull chin up by placing fingers behind the angles of the lower jaw and pushing forward.
- Take deep breath.
- Place your mouth over patient's nose *or* mouth, making leak-proof seal.
- If breathing into mouth, pinch patient's nostrils closed.
- If breathing into nose, seal patient's mouth with your hand.
- Blow into patient's nose or mouth until chest rises.
- Remove your mouth and let patient exhale.
- Repeat about 15 times a minute, or about every 4 seconds.
- If the patient's stomach rises markedly, exert moderate hand pressure on the stomach just below the rib cage to keep it from inflating.

For Infants:

- Place your mouth over patient's mouth *and* nose.
- Babies require only small puffs of air from your cheeks.
- Repeat 20 to 30 times per minute.
- Don't exaggerate the tilted position of an infant's head.

First Aid for Poisoning

In all cases, except poisonous bites, the principle is GET THE POISON OUT or OFF or DILUTE it. In the case of poisoning from plants, see chart on book pages 90-93. CALL PROMPTLY FOR EMERGENCY HELP.

Pages 174-176

SWALLOWED POISON

- Dilute poison by giving water, one or two glassfuls.
- Make patient vomit if so directed, BUT NOT IF:
  —patient is unconscious or having seizures.
  —swallowed poison was a strong corrosive (lye, strong acid, drain cleaner, etc.).
  —swallowed poison contains kerosene, gasoline or other petroleum distillates (unless containing a dangerous pesticide as well, which must be removed).

INDUCE VOMITING

- Give one tablespoonful (½ ounce) of syrup of ipecac for a child one year of age or older, plus at least one cup of water. If no vomiting occurs in 20 minutes, this dose may be repeated *once only*. After vomiting has ceased, offer a slurry of activated charcoal (1-2 tablespoonful) in a glass of water.
- If no ipecac syrup is available, try to induce vomiting by tickling back of throat with a spoon handle or other blunt object, after giving water. Do not give salt or mustard to children.
- Do not waste time waiting for vomiting, but transport patient promptly to a medical facility. *Bring package or container with intact label.*

INHALATION POISONING (Gas, Fumes, Smoke)

- Get into fresh clean air.
- Loosen clothing.
- If not breathing, start artificial respiration promptly. *Do not stop until breathing or help arrives.*
- Have *someone else* call for emergency help and transport to a medical facility promptly.

POISONOUS BITES

Snakes

- Don't let victim walk; keep as quiet as possible.
- Do not give alcohol.
- Call for emergency help and transport to a medical facility. *Enroute, or while awaiting transportation*
- Apply suction to bite wound with mouth or suction cup.
- If victim stops breathing use artificial respiration.

Insects

- Do not let victim walk; keep as quiet as possible.
- Place any available cold substance on bite area to relieve pain.
- A paste of Adolph's Meat Tenderizer or Baking Soda and water applied to the bite will often reduce the swelling and itching by its enzymatic action.
- If victim stops breathing, use artificial respiration.
- Call for emergency help and transport to a medical facility. (Persons with known unusual reactions to insect stings should carry emergency treatment kits and an emergency identity card).